LOCKDOWN

INDIA UNDER SIEGE FROM CORONA

SUNIL SHARAN

RosettaBooks®

NEW YORK 2020

First edition published 2020 by RosettaBooks

Cover design by Lon Kirschner

ISBN-13 (print): 978-0-7953-5299-7
ISBN-13 (ebook): 978-0-7953-5300-0

Library of Congress Control Number: 2020940709

RosettaBooks®

www.RosettaBooks.com

CONTENTS

CHAPTER ONE

MODI'S LOCKDOWN

*"Step outside in the next twenty-one days, and you set the
country back twenty-one years."*

—Prime Minister Modi on March 24, 2020

March 24, 2020, will go down as a seminal day in India's history. Indian prime minister Narendra Modi addressed the nation on TV and declared a national lockdown for three weeks. Modi had had fair warning. His favorite ally, the United States, had already put into place social distancing practices in most states, on March 20. So Modi had evidence regarding this virus, which was called by everyone from health-care professionals to politicians everything from tricky to vicious.

In one respect, at least, India was lucky. India had an approximate Patient Zero. On January 23, three medical students had traveled home to India from Wuhan, China. They had been studying at the Wuhan Institute of Medical Sciences and had been evacuated from China after the Chinese government announced it would lock down the city and other towns in Hubei Province because of the coronavirus. Back home in India, the students were quarantined and instructed to use disposable clothes, plates, and utensils.

But this was not the end of the story. On March 3, fifteen tourists from Italy were diagnosed with the virus and quarantined to a paramilitary camp of the Indo-Tibetan Police Force, and a forty-five-year-old man was diagnosed in Delhi, within the national capital region of India. Since the man's diagnosis, forty more people in Delhi had been diagnosed.

Things were nowhere near as grave a situation as that in the United States, but Modi knew he had work to do to keep it that way. On March 22, Modi declared a people's curfew. Many people took that to mean a holiday and took off on jaunts. Not so. Two days later, on March 24, Modi declared a lockdown for all of India.

Modi rarely smiles to Indians. The only time he lets his guard down is when he is with world leaders like Donald Trump, Xi Jinping, and Barack Obama. Trump visited India recently. He wrote in a commemorative book at Mahatma Gandhi's ashram that Modi was his dear friend. Then, in early April, he threatened "dear friend" Modi with retaliation if he wouldn't supply him with medicine for the coronavirus.

Modi cherishes his relationship with the US like no other country except perhaps Israel. He instantly agreed to supply the medication to the US. Then Trump hailed him, and Modi was happy. Modi has an uncanny ability to get along with world leaders. He was pals with the professorial Barack Obama. He is pals now with the mercurial Donald Trump. Angela Merkel of Germany has criticized Modi's policy in the Indian state of Kashmir. Modi has taken her criticism on the chin and has still welcomed her in India. Modi craves the acceptance of the world, partially because he had a rough ride getting to the top of India politics via the Hindu nationalist party the BJP, the political arm of the Hindu stormtrooper organization the RSS.

Now, Modi is known in India as the king of Hindu hearts. That is due in no small measure to the role he played in the horrific anti-Muslim riots in his state in 2002. In hindsight, his role seems to have been one more of omission than of commission, but Modi has received a hiding for what he did or did not do from India's left-wing media as well as from Indian National Congress president Sonia Gandhi.

Modi's international reputation was tarnished by the riots between Hindus and Muslims in 2002. The US and Europe banned him. He could only visit countries like Japan and China. But once he became the PM of India, Western countries were obliged to welcome him. And Modi knew that holding grudges would only hurt him and India. He embarked upon a campaign of hug diplomacy, greeting foreign leaders with a bear hug, and Modi started becoming popular in the West.

In Gujarat, Modi was known for his decisiveness. He carried the same decisiveness with him to the center. He instituted a couple of massive economic reforms, which backfired badly. His reputation as an economic genius lay in tatters. His base could not believe it. Modi would have lost the 2019 general elections had he not attacked Pakistan in retaliation for a terrorist attack it committed on Indian soil.

He romped home with a nearly two-thirds majority in Parliament. To amend the Constitution of India, you need a two-thirds majority in Parliament. Modi had it and duly amended the Constitution. He was as close to a dictator that India was going to get—a democratically elected dictator, but a dictator nevertheless.

Modi has visited China a number of times. He feels that the best way to deal with China is to kowtow to it. President Xi Jinping invited Modi to his home province of Wuhan a few years back. Modi is enamored of both China and the United States.

In Wuhan, where the coronavirus broke out, Xi instituted draconian measures to contain its spread. Modi watched and learned. The virus quickly spread to Europe and then to America. Modi followed Xi's example and imposed a complete lockdown in India. Indian epidemiologists like Dr. Ramanan Laxminarayan were calling only for a two-week lockdown, but Modi went a step further and instituted a three-week lockdown. It has now been extended until early May.

India had done very little testing, mostly on people returning from abroad. Modi knew that he could not get enough testing done in time to prevent a major outbreak. Lack of testing has been the bane in places like America, the UK, and Italy. Indians were shocked by Modi's decision to nearly quarantine the entire country when there had merely been a handful of deaths in the country and a few hundred cases detected.

Indians are notorious for their *chalta hai* (anything goes) attitude. The other thing Indians are famous for is *jugaad* (indigenous ingenuity). Modi doesn't believe in these fatalistic things. He didn't rise from being a boy selling tea barefoot on dirty railway platforms to becoming the ruler of the second-largest country in the world, and a man now feted in almost every world capital, by believing in fatalism.

Chalta hai and jugaad are attitudes that Modi has struggled with as PM. Gujaratis are relentless entrepreneurs. There are a million of them in America. About half the motels in the US and many hotels there are owned by them. Other Indians in general are much more laid-back. That's why despite a population of 1.3 billion fiercely fanatical about the game of cricket, a nation of just five million like New Zealand can thrash India's revered national cricket team.

Indians started getting stir-crazy a few days into the lockdown. The Indian doesn't do many outdoor activities like camping or canoeing or suchlike things. Unlike the American and the Brit, the Indian disdains running. Yet there are two outdoor things that an Indian likes to do.

One is playing cricket. Cricket can be played on a large field, where there is ample scope for social distancing. But Modi has banned field cricket as well. Cricket is more often played on the street, by rich and poor alike, often all together. Street cricket is much less demanding than field cricket, and players are much closer to one another. Taking street cricket away from the Indian is like taking candy away from a child. He will go bonkers!

The second outdoor activity that Indians indulge in is a brisk morning walk or a much more leisurely postprandial walk after dinner, often undertaken by couples, before they tuck in for some sex and sleep.

The favorite hobby of Indians is dropping by unannounced on friends and associates and spending hours gabbing and gossiping away. Cocktails and cards can also be on the table. It is very important for an Indian to mingle with her neighbors. It's not the kind of society like in America, where you can die alone in your apartment and no one will know for weeks.

Indians are nosy. It's almost like it's one big family partitioned off only by flimsy walls and gates. It's only the truly rich with their mansions who are immune from such prying eyes. But they have their own rich circles where everything about them is known. Modi lives alone in a majestic estate that dwarfs 10 Downing Street and even the White House. The mansion was formed by joining two massive colonial-era bungalows, 5 and 7 Racecourse Road. Number three Racecourse Road was then added. Modi didn't like the term "Racecourse," so he changed the name of his house to 7 Lok Kalyan Marg. *Lok Kalyan* means "welfare of the people." All of the welfare of the Indian people would thus flow from Modi's house. He is a bit of megalomaniac, isn't he?

Modi could feel that Indians were skittish about his lockdown. In a country of 1.4 billion, of course life is valued less than in a country of three hundred million or sixty million. But Hindus believe in reincarnation. This is absolutely central to the Hindu faith, that the soul never dies, that the body is just a garb.

I have asked my spiritual gurus where exactly the soul is, and they have struggled to answer. But if one life is going to lead to another, then the fear of loss of life becomes lesser. The fear of death becomes lesser.

In the Abrahamic religions, there is the concept of heaven and hell. In Hinduism, there are heaven and hell, too, but heaven is inhabited by celestial beings, like Indra, the god of rain. He is not really a god. The real aim of a Hindu is to reach the highest abode of Shri Krishna, Goluk, when he or she will be released from the constant cycle of birth and death.

To reach the abode of Krishna, Rama, or Shiva (take your pick) is the principal aim of Hindus. Of course Hindus can be reincarnated back to Earth or another earth planet.

That we are going somewhere after death dulls our sensitivity to death, and consequently to loss of life.

Modi also learned that health-care professionals were being harassed by their neighbors in case they had been infected by the virus. So he asked people to clang utensils in support of doctors and nurses. How that might have helped, I don't know. He should have asked his cops to arrest the offending parties, but I guess he didn't want to seem sterner than he was already seeming.

The lockdown in India is unlike the one in the US. No planes fly, and no trains or buses are running. State governors obey without question Modi's diktats, even though India is as federal a democracy as America is.

No state governor is eager to take advantage of the crisis to become PM, as you see some doing in the US. Sure, Andrew Cuomo in New York gives good press briefings, and his virus-infected brother, Chris Cuomo of CNN, is building him up to run for president, and sure Gretchen Whitmer of Michigan is attractive and taking the president head-on and quite possibly likely to become Joe Biden's running mate, but don't they run two of the most virus-afflicted states in the country? What does that say about the level of pandemic preparedness of they themselves and of their states? America, I will never understand you.

Indian industry, like Germany, is heavily oriented toward small and medium enterprises. Many don't take a day off the whole year. It's sacrilegious for them to stay shut, but stay shuttered they are. Modi, though, has the trust of the people. They believe him. They believe in him. He is India's pied piper. Wherever he wants to take them, they will follow.

Modi is absolutely determined that India not become a Wuhan or a Europe or America. But people are starving and he will have to ease up soon. His government so far has done well in distributing food to the poor and needy, but how long governmental reserves and resolve last remains to be seen.

Also, community spreading has already taken hold in India. If and when Modi opens up, there could be an unmanageable spike in cases. Will he put the shutters down again? Modi consults with very few as he takes major decisions. He is single and lives alone and so has no one even in his personal life to confide to. His most important confidant is India's erratic and ill-qualified home minister, Amit Shah, also from Modi's state of Gujarat, whose bumbling ways have often gotten Modi into hot water.

Modi wants to rule India for another ten to fifteen years. To lock down more or not to—that is the question that Modi is fast coming up against. His fate depends upon whether he gets the answer mostly right. According to the data generated by the Indian government's premier policy think tank, NITI Aayog, if a lockdown had not been implemented, India would have witnessed over 1,022,283 active COVID cases. As of May 15, 2020, India had 85,856 active COVID cases and 2,746 deaths from the virus. That's a death rate of 3.20 percent. If a lockdown had not been implemented,

India would have seen 32,713 deaths from the virus. So far, so good. But this was only the beginning, and with only four hours to catch a bus or a train home between the announcement of the lockdown and its beginning, many Indian workers were left stranded. And none of the wealthy were donating bus service or a private plane to ferry them home.

CHAPTER TWO

MAN WITH THE MIDAS TOUCH?

The train from Ahmedabad approaches the town of Vadnagar in the Indian state of Gujarat twice a day. Vadnagar has only one platform. The train is slow, for the gauge of the tracks is narrow. The train only has second-class and third-class compartments, and like everything in India, it is packed to the gills.

The train will stop in Vadnagar for five minutes. There is one tea stall in the station. It is owned and operated by Damodardas Mulchand Modi. He has six children. The third is a boy called Narendra Damodardas Modi. This boy is very agile, so when he is six, his father ropes him in to help with the tea stall. The boy, laden with clay cups filled with tea, climbs the train as it approaches the station and then run across from one compartment to another selling his tea. Some people pay him immediately, while others want to pay later.

Modi was Gujarat's governor from 2001 to 2014, and he spent this time with only one goal in mind: how to ascend the throne of Delhi. His stint in the mountains, a time he does not dwell on much, seems to have turned Modi's will into iron. He ran Gujarat like a virtual dictator. He was voted the best governor of India a number of times. He roped in many industrialists like Mukesh Ambani, himself a Gujarati, to his cause. In one's bid to become the supreme leader of the land, it always helps to have moneybags on your side, for they are the ones who subsidize India's ridiculously expensive elections.

If you win, in return you reward your pals with crony contracts. That's how 131 "dollar billionaires" have been minted in India since 1991. Think for a second. Can you think of a single world-famous Indian product? A car? A phone? A plane? Yes, there are companies peddling software programmers. And there is yoga, but no Indian company is making money out of it (in contrast, a Canadian company called Lululemon has made millions out of yoga gear and wear). The reason Indian companies are unable to generate world-class products is because they are in the main part run by crony capitalists.

But it is not only Modi who has capitalists as his cronies. The Congress has them. Every political party in India has them. The whole economy of the country is being hollowed out by these parasites, these termites, but nobody wants to do anything about it. Sonia Gandhi's government collapsed in 2014 in a miasma of crony capitalism, but those capitalists just transferred their skills to Modi, who became PM that same year.

Modi generated double-digit economic growth most years that he was the governor of Gujarat. He brought in loads of foreign investment. India's growth from 1947 (independence from the British) until 1991 (when countrywide economic reforms were unleashed) was an anemic 4 percent on an annual basis. This growth rate got dubbed the Hindu rate of growth, which implied that Hindus could never grow more than 4 percent.

The alarming thing was that India's population was galloping along in what came to be known as a population explosion. India has tried to curb its population growth, but without much success. Economists believe that the only way India will get rid of dire economic poverty and become something of a middle-income country is if it reaches growth figures in almost double digits.

Modi ran his 2014 election campaign for prime ministership with customary élan. The style of shirt that he wore came to be known as the Modi Shirt. He had holograms of himself all over the country drawing in the faithful and even the not so faithful. He hired a battery of Muslim spokesmen and women to espouse his cause and neutralize his anti-Muslim image. The wildly popular Muslim Bollywood star Salman Khan endorsed him. Khan had government cases against him, but when Modi came to power, they were conveniently dismissed.

It was a landslide victory in 2014. Modi won an absolute (more than 50 percent) majority in Parliament. Sonia Gandhi's Congress party was nearly wiped out, retaining less than 8 percent of the seats. Now she would have to face her "merchant of death"—which is what she called Modi after the bloody riots in the Indian state of Gujarat in 2002—every day in Parliament, except that she would be seated on the opposition benches and he on the treasury. For five long years.

Modi was new to Delhi. Delhi is like Washington, DC, a city of palace intrigue and power brokers and schemers and outright thieves. One has to know one's way around. One has to know the right people. Modi hired an old Delhi hand, Arun Jaitley, as both his finance minister as well as defense minister. Jaitley would take care of Delhi for Modi.

For more than fifty years, India's notorious bureaucracy, the Indian Administrative Service, which was in effect the real ruler of the country, had served the Nehru-Gandhi family. Many owed their entire career, their entire existence to the family. Suck up to the family and you could go far. Cross the family, and you were toast. Neither Nehru nor Indira nor Rajiv nor Sonia—the four Nehru-Gandhi rulers—had any compunction in rewarding praise and punishing calumny. How would the bureaucracy react to an interloper like Modi?

And the media? Many right-wingers had supported Modi and would obviously be rewarded with plum assignments. But what about the vast left-wing media, much of it in hock to the Gandhi family? Six years of Modi, and the struggle continues. India's media is polarized about Modi. Indian prime ministers are expected to address the media every now and then, if only on planes when flying abroad. Modi hasn't given a single press conference to Indian media—not on the ground, not in the air. He doesn't want the riots of 2002 to be raked up. Let the past bury its dead.

A couple of years into his time as PM, the economy was not really looking up. Modi started developing itchy fingers; he had to do something to prove that he was an economic genius. He decided to demonetize all high-currency notes because he felt they led to the circulation of black money (money on which income tax had not been paid). There was a mad scramble all over India to return these high-currency notes and obtain lower-currency ones. There were miles-long lines. People poked and prodded, jostled and squabbled. People died in the searing heat. Demonetization crippled the economy because much of the Indian economy is run on cash transactions of black money. Modi insisted that what he had done was correct despite all evidence to the contrary. It is only now that he has stopped touting up demonetization.

Another major reform was long overdue, a standardization of the sales tax structure throughout the country. Modi launched his goods and services tax with great fanfare, but it was implemented hastily and haphazardly and led to great consternation within the people. Was Modi losing his Midas touch, people wondered?

General elections were due in 2019. Modi was flailing. Luckily for him, his opposition was flailing, too. But there was every chance that Modi would lose. And then Pakistan launched a jihadi attack on Indian soil. In previous such occurrences, Indian prime ministers had failed to retaliate overtly against Pakistan for fear of full-scale nuclear war breaking out in the subcontinent. But not so Modi. He kept Pakistan in suspense for ten days and then launched a potent and patently visible air strike in Pakistan. Pakistan stood humiliated; Indians were elated. India's eternal enemy had been humbled. Modi romped home with ease in the general elections.

But India's economy was still struggling. Modi couldn't get it back on track. The real problem was that Modi's BJP party lacked financial whiz kids. Modi had inherited some from the previous Congress's administration, like the former IMF chief economist Raghuram Rajan. Modi himself brought in another economic expert, the Columbia professor Arvind Panagriya, to India, but westernized people like Rajan and Panagriya didn't fit into the BJP's homegrown culture and were forced to leave. None of Modi's ministers are economic experts. None of his bureaucrats are. He has been left twiddling his thumbs over the economy. The man definitely seemed to have lost his Midas touch.

That his economy was cantering at a tepid 4 percent while the whole world had thought that he would make it gallop at 10 percent was galling to Modi. He had to do something, but he didn't know what. He could ask the westernized Indian experts to come back to India and help him, and they would, but that would be like losing face for himself and his lackeys within his party, which would mean pretty much the entire party itself.

Modi did not want to waste his landslide victory. Indian voters are notoriously fickle and turn upon you if their expectations are not met. Modi was not going to be able to meet their economic expectations. He turned his attention toward the Indian state of Kashmir and consolidated his hold over it. Indian Kashmir's population is about thirteen million. Long before the coronavirus lockdown, Modi put the entire state of Kashmir under a strict curfew in August 2019, and that too without any internet access. He thus gained some experience of what a lockdown entails. The Kashmir lockdown is ongoing.

Modi's actions in Kashmir met with fierce resistance from Pakistan, which claimed the Muslim-majority state as its own. Pakistan blew hot, it blew cold, but it knew that until the Afghan endgame ended and it was able to direct jihadis from there into Kashmir, it could do nothing. Modi had once again bested Pakistan. His base was delirious.

Soon thereafter, in December 2019, Modi invited religious minorities—Hindus, Sikhs, Christians, Buddhists, Jains, and Parsis—from the Muslim states of Pakistan, Bangladesh, and Afghanistan to immigrate to India. There is no doubt that these minorities are heavily persecuted in these countries. Hindus, Sikhs, Jains, and Buddhists belong to Indic religions, and it is natural that India would offer solace to followers of these faiths. India has given refuge to Parsis for twelve hundred years, and they are very small in number. It is the inclusion of Christians that is interesting. Christians number about four million in Pakistan and are highly oppressed. But in India, too, they are often seen askance, as puppets of the West. Modi's party, the BJP, has been accused of instigating violence against them and vandalizing their places of worship. Why then the sudden love for Christians in Modi's heart?

Well, including Christians in the list would make the whole project palatable to the West, which is something that Modi deeply cares about. Missing notably from the list were Muslims. Incredibly enough, Muslims are persecuted in Pakistan, Bangladesh, and Afghanistan. In Pakistan, the Muslim Shia minority often faces violence at the hands of the Sunni majority. Another Muslim sect, the Ahmaddiyas, are seen as deviants and heavily discriminated against. And then if Modi wanted to make India as a haven for the world's persecuted, why didn't he invite one of the most oppressed people in the world, and that too living in his neighborhood, the Muslim Rohingyas of Myanmar, to come to India?

The message was clear—Muslims were not welcome in India. India's two hundred million–strong Muslim minority went into an uproar. The nation came to a standstill. Many liberal Hindu Indians supported India's Muslims. Donald Trump visited Delhi. On the exact day of his visit, ten miles from where he was being serenaded by Modi, Hindu-Muslim riots broke out in which one hundred people perished. Modi had egg on his face.

Coronavirus came to his rescue. He locked the country down on March 24, first for three weeks. Kashmir had already been in lockdown mode for close to seven months. Now the rest of the country would experience what the people of Kashmir had been experiencing. India is an interesting country. Hindus and Muslims in India are in general solipsistic. In Kashmir, the Muslim majority mercilessly ethnically cleansed Hindus from the state. In return, the state of India persecuted Kashmiri Muslims. But the Hindus in the rest of India felt nothing for the Muslims of Kashmir. In fact, when Kashmir was placed under curfew, many Hindus were happy because they felt that Kashmiri Muslims had it coming to them.

Now those very Hindus are under lockdown, and yes, they care about it. Indian media is full of stories of celebrities coping with the lockdown, of the middle class furious at being clamped indoors, and of the suffering of the poor. All of this within days of Modi's lockdown starting, but when he imposed the curfew in Kashmir, there was a nary a peep from India's chatterati. Indians believe that Kashmir belongs to them, but when the Indian state imposes suffering on Kashmiri Muslims, the just shrug their shoulders and say that the Muslims of Kashmir deserve the treatment because of what they had done to the Hindus of Kashmir.

Modi once again became India's messiah. The Muslim demonstrations against the flawed immigration bill were rudely dismissed. Modi regularly appeared on TV asking Indians to stand as one against the virus. Funny— sometimes he seems to divide Indians, and then he seeks to unite them. He begged forgiveness from India's poor for the suffering imposed on them. Unlike in the US, Modi did not constitute a visible task force. He was the very visible superman combating the virus alone. Once Modi's cabinet appeared behind him on TV, all seated at desks like they have at school, with six feet of social distancing separating them, but they seemed like errant schoolboys under the tutelage of Modi. They never again appeared on TV like that. Combating corona has been a Modi show all the way.

People in India are tiring of Modi's propaganda-like speeches. But he's India's pied piper now; they just have to follow him. Modi for now has confronted the virus early. Modi hasn't had many deaths this first time round, but because he's been conducting next-to-nil testing within the country, he risks a huge spike in cases if he lifts the lockdown.

Such then are the perils that men with the Midas touch face. They can't always turn economies into gold. By the same token, can they prevent them from turning into dust?

CHAPTER THREE

THE RICH MAN'S MADE IT

The Australian cricket team has an anthem they chant every time they win, which, to the consternation of the rest of the cricket world, is often and almost always. It is politically incorrect, but I'll say it here: "Australia, You Fuckin' Beauty." It is an ode to a country created by convicts and their descendants by practically wiping out indigenous populations. It is a beautiful land, is Australia—a fuckin' beauty.

India, too, like Australia, is a vast and varied land, perhaps even more beautiful. Australia lacks the majestic Himalayas; the tigers roaming around in forests; the gigantic rivers, the Ganges and the Brahmaputra; the beauty of Kashmir and Kerala; and of women of varying hues, all imbued with a stunning allure. And yes, Australia lacks Bollywood. But Australia and India have one thing in common, and that is cricket. And Australia has arguably the better cricket team. The better batsmen and the better bowlers, fast or spin. It is inconceivable that the Aussies would have a better spin bowler than the Indians, but there you are. Indians want nothing more than to trample upon the corpse of the Australian cricket team. So that the motto of their cricket team too can be India, You Fuckin' Beauty.

But that motto cannot be for all Indians, at least for nearly a billion that struggle and starve every day. That motto is reserved for India's rich, who enjoy seeing themselves as a breed apart.

An Indian billionaire driving his own car and a modest one? Inconceivable! As inconceivable as the earth being flat. Actually, that is more conceivable. The only people who really and truthfully can chant "India, You Fuckin' Beauty" are the Indian rich. They are a breed like none other; they lead a life like no other. They can go through an entire life without lifting a finger. Actually, just by lifting their pinkie, they have the whole world at their beck and call.

They have never cooked a dish in all their lives, never cleaned a robe, never washed a piece of cloth, never ironed anything, never shined shoes, never driven a car. Cleaning the toilet bowl? Nah, they would die a thousand deaths.

It's hard to put a figure on the exact number of India's truly rich. India has generated 131 dollar billionaires since 1991. Ah, to be a dollar billionaire in India. Every Indian's dream! Only the US and China, in that order, have more dollar billionaires than India. And the Indian dollar billionaires, they are billionaires in real-dollar terms, not in some funky purchasing parity way. Multiply every dollar by seventy, which is what one dollar is worth in Indian rupees in real exchange terms, and you can imagine how rich these billionaires are in Indian terms. Now apply purchasing power parity, and you will realize that each Indian dollar billionaire is about four times richer than his US counterpart with the same number of dollars.

But the dollar billionaires are the über-rich. There are many other rich people in India. All in all, there are about twenty million people in India who are truly rich.

These twenty million people lead a lifestyle that billionaires in the US do not lead, that the sheikhs of Arabia perhaps lead. Waited on hand and foot, they can travel to wherever they want and do whatever they want. They often get away with murder, even in plain sight.

The rich wanted Modi to do one thing for them: make them even richer. The billionaires wanted to become multibillionaires, the millionaires billionaires. Along the way, Modi realized that to get to the top he would have to strike bargains with the rich. After all, who else would fund his expensive electoral campaigns and his scorched-earth demolition jobs of the opposition?

A pandemic is a great equalizer. The virus has no idea what or whom it infects. The virus is colorblind, but money can help when it comes to "disease distancing"—a term being used in India in lieu of "social distancing," which can be seen as prejudicial toward those of the lower castes in the Hindu religion. The rich close their doors and isolate in luxury. Now, what the wealthy in India want from Modi is to keep them, if not immune, exempt. While the truly rich in India have lost all ability to use their hands and feet to do chores like cooking and cleaning, they will learn. Bereft of domestic help during the pandemic, they are truly lost. Katrina Kaif, a famous Bollywood actress, exemplified this on the first day of the lockdown. She posted videos of herself cleaning dishes and sweeping floors. It was obvious that she was brand-new to all this, and it was completely hilarious. I am sure Kaif posted her pictures to generate a few laughs. I didn't understand what was so funny and wrote an article in the *Times of India* called "What's so funny, India?"

Another actress, Priyanka Chopra, who has married the American singer Nick Jonas, eleven years her junior, couldn't resist French-kissing him, as captured by a website, not realizing that saliva is the primary way in which the virus spreads. The website, of course, kept the picture up for days on end, all at the onset of the lockdown in India. Websites and other publications have sprung up, ready to post all the antics of the bold and the beautiful. It's well-nigh impossible for a TV channel or a website to abstain from pandering to the stars, for there are so many other media outlets ready to cheapen themselves. So join the gang one must.

India is obsessed with celebrities, and what better way is there for celebrity publications and TV channels to garner clickbait or TV ratings than to feed into this obsession? Nobody can discipline the celebs, though. Nobody wants to discipline the celebs. Not only are they über-rich, but they are extremely powerful as well. If gods walk upon this earth, then it is they, Indian film stars and cricket stars. They are at the apex of India's glitterati. Politicians tremble at their fan following and try desperately to be become popular by association.

There are film stars and cricket stars who have killed people in broad daylight but strut around India without an inkling of any fear. Their murderous antics have only added to their lore. Poorer classes see them get away scot-free with murder, and wish, *Oh, if it only was us.* So the aspiration builds up from bottom to top, an aspiration not only for money and the comforts money brings, but also for power and immunity from justice. All of it makes for a very aspirational country. But with the economy growing at the sclerotic rate of about 3 percent (for a developing country) before the onset of the pandemic, a growth rate that promises to career to near zero for at least one year, nobody from any poor class is ascending.

In fact a lot of rich people will fall down a notch or two, something absolutely galling to them. They will not be able to buy that new Tesla, or invest in a farmhouse, or ask their stockbroker to do insider trading for them (insider trading is rampant in India and seems to go on virtually without any impunity). The über-rich have also stashed away mounds of money in tax havens abroad, so they will be carry on their ostentatious lifestyles, but the shoes of the rich, who are a clear notch below the über-rich, will start showing signs of wear and tear.

The Indian government is testing and quarantining for a period of fourteen days anyone who returns from abroad. One rich lady in my, if I may say so, rather posh neighborhood was told that a couple of foreigners had come to India and were staying in her building. Petrified, she proceeded to sterilize all of the stairwells, including the banisters. The rich in India know that they have a rich life. An entitled life. A privileged life. They have the best of both worlds in India—Western brands and Indian lifestyle. They are la crème de la crème. They don't want to die. They will do anything not to die. The finest medical care—at a price—is available to them in India. And if Indian doctors cannot fix them up, they can always fly abroad.

The rich in India have huge houses and therefore are not going as stir-crazy in the lockdown as the middle classes. Their houses are replete with lawns and gardens, although swimming pools tend to be the preserve of only the superrich because of the maintenance required, especially in India's hot, dusty, and polluted climate. Edwin Lutyens was a British architect who built New Delhi for the British to stay in before India became independent from the British. Today, what is known as Lutyens' Delhi, which is where Prime Minister Modi lives, counts among the most expensive residential real estate anywhere in the world.

Lutyens' Delhi is replete with colonial-era bungalows, which do not seem to have changed an iota since independence from the British. Here India's power elite stays: ministers and other top politicians, the high judiciary, the military top brass, senior bureaucrats, and a few industrialists. It is so exclusive that it even though it is located in the city of Delhi, a municipality separate from Delhi's manages it. Each house has a lawn that is so large that it can be used as a running track. It is the poor for whom density is a problem. It is easy for the superrich to keep their distance in the lap of luxury.

COVID doesn't strike here. There is ample room for social distancing. One should note that hardly any rich person in India has been struck by COVID. Modi's lockdown has succeeded in stopping a rampage that has been seen in the United States and Europe. But if you don't test adequately, you don't know who is infected and whom to isolate, whom to follow for contact tracing. The other question is of immunity. It is unclear what sort of immunity through antibodies occurs in an infected person. But let's assume that some sort of immunity develops. With extreme social distance as practiced by Modi, the majority of the population may not get infected, but then it does not develop any immunity. When social distancing is lifted, as it must inevitably, nonimmune people will perforce come in contact with infected people, with the concomitant risk of large-scale community transmission. Dr. Ashish Jah of the Harvard Global Health Institute has likened the pandemic to that other bat-and-ball sport, baseball, stating, "If this were a baseball game, it would be the second inning, and there's no reason to think that by the ninth inning the rest of the world that looks now like it hasn't been affected won't become like other places." The rich can afford to watch the game play out from a distance, if not to leave the stadium.

If community transmission develops rapidly after the lockdown is lifted, many of the gains of the lockdown would be lost. But the rich would be immune to all this. They are very cognizant of what is going on in the West, especially the States. If people in the States have started wearing masks, albeit belatedly, they will start wearing masks. The rich will get tested. They will get their domestic help and even staff members tested. So, all their drivers and cooks and sweepers and gardeners and butlers will have to traipse to the testing booth. Testing may not be available for India's poor, but for the rich anything can be arranged.

A rapid test has been developed by Abbott Laboratories of the United States, but they are busy coping with the rampant demand in their own country, so just forget about making it available to countries like India.

So how is all of this pertinent to India's rich? Well, everything that happens in the West is pertinent to India's rich. The rich and the über-rich have extensive business dealings with the West. They follow intimately what is going on in the West. Priyanka Chopra and Nick Jonas are feted by India's elite. Even the prime minister, who hardly attends social functions, made it a point to attend their wedding reception.

Another top actress and cricket team owner, Preity Zinta, married her American financier beau Gene Goodenough and even moved to the States. Australian cricketers came to play cricket in India and picked up Indian wives in the bargain.

India's elite knows that life in the West is not that easy; they know that they have *la dolce vita* sitting right here in India. They are not going to trade it for any other life. Certainly not for death. Medical experts the world over, including in India, are cautioning that the pandemic could go on and on for a couple of years. Stop social distancing, infected cases spike again, then begin a lockdown once again, and so on and so forth.

If the pandemic had not struck the West, the rich of India would have safely decamped to Western shores. But the West is under siege. As of now at least India is a safer bet than the West. So, India's dollar billionaires and millionaires are staying put in India. Six hundred people serve Mukesh Ambani and his family in the billion-dollar home, Antilia, that he has constructed for himself in Mumbai. It's the world's most expensive private residence after Buckingham Palace. It's got three helipads and a swimming pool floating in the sky. It should have looked classy, but instead it appears like a hotchpotch of matchboxes stacked one on top of another, with the whole structure seeming to tilt over at any moment. I wouldn't

want to live there, but there Ambani lives with his large family and a reti-
nue of six hundred servants. It's impossible to maintain social distancing
in such a milieu, especially since the staff is supposed to wait hand and
foot upon you at close quarters.

I am sure the entire staff is getting tested for COVID at regular inter-
vals. The Ambani life is repeated across India in the mansions of many
billionaires and millionaires. Their lives are extremely precious, so their
servants have to be clean. They have the heft to call any minister and ask to
jump the queue for testing. I wouldn't mind being a personal servant of a
dollar billionaire in India. At least I would know that my life is in good
hands. For the superrich and the rich of India, the pandemic is still a cozy
catastrophe, a legitimate horror viewed from their still very safe distance.

The actor Kamal Haasan, a megastar, has criticized Modi's lockdown.
He says that the rich build their lives on the backs of the poor. Haasan has
just started a political party and seems to be aiming to gain brownie points
with the poor—while poor they might be, nevertheless they vote in large
numbers in elections. Me thinks that thou protest too much, Mr. Haasan.
Of course he ends his tirade against the PM by saying that he's on his side.
Why? Well, you never know. Modi just might make him a minister.

CHAPTER FOUR

CAUGHT IN THE MUDDLE

My grandfather who died in the 1960s was fluent in Persian, which was still the language of the courts. It's only the Hindu generation of today that has lost touch with Persian. The Hindus had their own languages—Sanskrit and Hindi—but reserved them for private use. The British in the nineteenth century had sought to stamp out both Sanskrit and Persian (and their bodies of literature) in favor of English.

In the Hindu caste system, there are four classes, with the Brahmins at the top and warriors occupying the second tier. The king came from the warrior caste. It is instructive to note that the king is placed below the Brahmins, although of course his writ over the kingdom is supreme. The Brahmins are learned monks, well versed in Hindu scriptures, of which there are a gazillion, and some of whom serve as advisers to the king. It is important to note the stress Hinduism places on learning; it is central to the faith. In no other faith will you perhaps find as much of an emphasis on learning as in Hinduism.

Even the Indian untouchable class, which was sent to faraway lands by the British as indentured labor, cling to education as their savior. So in Trinidad you have Indians outdoing the native population in all aspects of learning; it is the same with the Indians of Fiji and the Samoans there. All across Africa, there are Indians teaching in a wide variety of schools. I cannot tell you the number of Kenyans who have come up to me and said that their schoolteacher was Indian.

Buried so far away from their native land, in a foreign land so strange and anarchic, these graves tell tales of conquerors and racists and bigots, sometimes softened by noblesse oblige and kindness.

India is a poor country. If you are fat, you are labeled healthy. People say that you belong to a prosperous house, one in which there is enough to eat and drink. The poor of India are desperate to belong to such houses, but sadly that is not their fate. The poor in India are in general thin and wiry. I have lived in France and was shocked at how tiny the portions there were compared to America. But when you have an exodus of poverty from the old continent to the new one, what do poor people crave most? It is food. So, they eat, and they eat, and as a European told my father at Disney World in Florida, the average American bloats after age twenty-five.

So, what has this got to do with the coronavirus? The poor in India tend to be fit—not so the United States. Obesity is an underlying condition that can increase the risk for contracting the coronavirus.

The US is about three times the physical size of India, and the US has almost a billion fewer citizens. As of May 15, the US has recorded more than eighty thousand deaths, before India's death toll hit two thousand. There are many issues that must factor into any comparison of these numbers. The virus is a work in progress worldwide; nobody knows what's to come. Even scientists are using the word *luck*.

Testing is only now becoming widespread in India, though India was early to take the temperature of those arriving by plane from other countries. Even with the largest confinement ever attempted in human history, India's infection rate continued to rise.

Despite the incomplete data, it must be said that the rate of infection in India is at this point lower than that in the West. Metropolises like New York, Paris, and London have been devastated, while teeming New Delhi has, so far, largely been spared. Yet the Western press looks toward India, too often, as falling short and soon to be under siege by the virus. Why?

Scientists are studying this phenomenon. Journalists need to do more extensive reporting on what is so far a medical anomaly.

The one hundred million–strong English-speaking middle class constitutes what is called India's chatterati. It is what the English-speaking media says that determines policy in India. I write for the *Times of India*, the world's most popular English-speaking daily, which has a daily reach of about twenty million. The Times Group, of which the *Times of India* is part, and which includes its numerous other papers and magazines and websites, has a daily reach of four hundred million people. Just imagine that! A daily reach bigger than the population of the US and equal about to the population of the European Union.

Yet the Indian middle class is very sensitive to anything negative written about India in Western papers, all of whose reach is much smaller than the *Times of India*. You will never, ever see a positive article about India in Western papers like the *New York Times* and the *Guardian*. The best way for an Indian author to get published in these papers is to indulge in India-bashing—a relatively obscure Indian journalist named Pragya Tiwari wrote an op-ed on March 25, 2020, in the *New York* Times decrying India's efforts in combating the coronavirus.

The same issues that she highlighted—lack of testing, lack of personal protective equipment, lack of social distancing, lack of food security for the poor—were much more amply present in the US.

Tiwari failed to mention that when the virus struck Hubei Province in China, PM Modi sent tons and tons of emergency medical equipment like masks and gloves to China. Modi never blames China for the spread of the virus. And when Modi felt that there was a danger to his country, he locked his country down.

Wherever you go in the US, you will see many Americans not wearing masks. I haven't seen a single American leader appearing on TV or otherwise wearing a mask. PM Modi just addressed the nation wearing a mask, with his entire team behind him wearing masks. Wearing a thirty-cent mask is in actuality the safest and most practical way to practice social distancing. Indians cannot leave their houses for a stroll or to visit friends and indulge in gossip, their favorite pastime. They cannot play cricket, golf, or cards. All eating establishments are closed. There is no takeout or delivery. Cook whatever you want at home. Is there any wonder that with such tough regulations, deaths have so far been modest?

But the Indian middle class is chafing at the bit. It wants release from the shackles that Modi has put it under. The middle class in India has one and only aspiration, which is to break into the rich class. From a small house to a big house, from a small car to a luxury car, from a simple wedding to a big fat Indian wedding, that's what the Indian middle class lives for.

That's why all the world's brands have made a beeline toward India. India today risks becoming a colony once again. It exports mainly raw material and human labor and imports all kinds of finished goods. Gandhi must be turning in his grave. All that fasting unto death to not remain a colony, all that torture seemingly for nothing.

The middle class is not as spoiled as the rich class. If the rich class—the actors, the industrialists, the cricket stars—are the glitterati, the English-speaking middle class—the managers, the engineers, the doctors, the lawyers—are the chatterati. It is outnumbered by the poor, but it defines public opinion in India.

Much of the middle class has domestic help in some shape or form. Perhaps the women have an assistant who will help them cut and clean in the kitchen, unlike the rich class, where it would be heresy if the housewife would deign to enter the kitchen. The rich all have a chauffeur or even many chauffeurs to drive them around. The middle class may not be able to afford a chauffeur. The rich, of course, depend upon the poor, but they also depend upon the middle class for their prosperity. Who would run a rich industrialist's business if not middle-class managers?

Who would minister to the rich if not middle-class doctors? It must be said that often enough doctors in India are not middle class but can be rich just like in the US. Who would plead for the rich if not middle-class lawyers? Much of the middle class is what is called service class in India (as opposed to the rich business class) and lives from paycheck to paycheck. Of course the middle class saves for a daughter's wedding or a son's education or a nest egg for their own retirement, but that money is not supposed to be touched for everyday expenditure.

The rich have oodles of money in umpteen safe havens; the middle class doesn't. The middle class wants the lockdown to end. Sure, it doesn't mind doing the washing and the cooking and cleaning for a while, but it doesn't want the economy to grind to a halt and then be forced to break its nest eggs. Modi came to power in 2014 and promised double-digit growth. For most of his first term in office, from 2014 to 2019, he has given only half that.

The middle class lost confidence in the previous prime minister, Manmohan Singh, because his government got embroiled in corruption, but Singh gave the country a consistent 8 percent growth rate for ten years. There is nostalgia for Singh now; there is incredulity that Modi has not performed on the economic front. If the growth rate doesn't ramp up, the middle class will not move into the rich class. With the virus and the lockdown, growth is on the skids and may end up almost zero for the year.

This is a nightmarish scenario for the middle class. Even with the lockdown, community transmission has definitely arrived in India. State governors (known in India as chief ministers) have extended all support to Modi as he has extended the lockdown. But the middle class has had enough of it.

It lives for the most part in cramped quarters in cities such as Mumbai and Delhi with some of the highest real-estate prices in the world. Not in the ample bungalows and big houses that the rich are used to. The middle-class is going stir-crazy. The men are learning to cook, but they have never stepped into a kitchen before, so they are not doing all that well. They are trying to clean but end up dirtying everything.

As everywhere, the kids are at home all the time. For couples, there are few, if any, date nights. India's middle class chatters a lot in the office; it can put in long hours but is nowhere as productive as the Germans or the South Koreans.

Working from home is an alien concept in India. At home, there is the distraction of TV, films, music, family. The Indian middle class is not disciplined enough to work from home. If a man doesn't go to an office in India, he is considered to be not working.

The middle class wants out of the lockdown. The middle class will force Modi to open up his shutters sooner than later. Their pockets are hurting, their minds are turning senile, their libidos are febrile. All of the gains of Modi's lockdown stand to be undone because of the intransigence of the middle class and their inability to abide by the rules of the lockdown.

CHAPTER FIVE

THE POOR MAN'S BUST

Smarajit Jana, a public health scientist in Kolkata, has said the one-size-fits-all strategy of the lockdown is likely to fail. In Kolkata alone, 40 percent of residents live in slums where often four individuals share one room of approximately seven square feet. Under such circumstances, any kind of distancing is worse than a cruel joke. Recently, in three slums in Mumbai, where conditions are just as dire, more people have tested positive for COVID-19. And this is after the lockdown had been put in place. Inevitably, the virus has now escaped into the general community.

The migrant workers are also suffering, crowded into small places, with little chance of keeping even two feet of distance from each other. Many are stranded at city borders because the lockdown only allowed four hours for people to manage to shelter in place before all public transportation was literally shut down. And the "safe houses" allotted to them are anything but safe. Once again, they are many to a room, making disease distancing impossible. The quarters are unhygienic. There are flies. What plumbing there is often doesn't work, contributing to the unsanitary conditions.

A single twenty-second hand wash uses more than half a gallon of water. The average American household uses one hundred gallons of water per day. Washing your hands all day in the United States is clearly a cinch. Not so in India. According to the April 7 issue of *National Geographic*, only one-fifth of Indian households have running water. Government water tank trucks are now delivering to villages twenty to twenty-five liters of water per day, which would be enough for the requisite hand washings if no water was needed for anything else. But often, the water trucks don't show up. This is a lose/lose situation.

In addition, many Indian cities have red light districts, including Kolkata and Mumbai. More than five thousand sex workers live in the Sonagachi area of Kolkata. Once again living conditions—one family, one room—make keeping your distance an impossibility. Finally, between 15 and 20 percent of the populations of Mumbai and Kolkata, including children, live on the street. These people are not only vulnerable to the virus but also fall into the realm of the underreported. According to Reuters, with hundreds of millions of poor Indians living in unhygienic and crammed-in conditions, there is a very real fear that if the testing starts too far behind the curve, the confirmed cases won't even account for the tip of the tip of the iceberg. One would have to be naive to believe India's official numbers on the virus. At the very least, they do not include the numbers of those who died recently of sudden pneumonia without being tested. Former finance minister and a leader of the opposition party P. Chidambaram has said, "There is unanimity among epidemiologists, doctors, and district-level administrators that the need of the hour is aggressive and extensive testing."

Yet any campaign for massive testing is hampered by a lack of test kits and lack of personal protective equipment.

Modi has allocated over $400 million from his PM CARES Fund as of May 2020. That same month, Modi also announced a $260 billion relief package for India's $3 trillion economy. He was scant about the details. All of these belated actions and announcements affect India's working poor, for whom life has never been easy.

India has a long history of the superrich and the superpoor. Textbooks in Indian schools often refer to India as "The Golden Sparrow." Historically, India has been a storehouse for the world's gold, but its defensive strategy was like that of a sparrow, founded on nonaggression. No wonder India was plundered again and again.

If India was a golden sparrow during the time of the great Mughals, then that sparrow seemed to squawk only for the king and nobles and perhaps some in the merchant class. The rest of the populace was dirt poor. In a famous picture, Jehangir, that most Indian-looking of the great Mughals, is shown as taking a bow and arrow to a black ghoul. The ghoul represents poverty in India. Precisely four centuries after Jehangir, and innumerable rulers after him, the ghoul of Indian poverty is still alive and kicking.

Indian poverty has remained endemic, and Indian rulers have been unable to do anything about it. About a quarter-century ago, poverty was assumed if a household earned less than a dollar a day. That ridiculously low figure was later upped to two dollars a day. Two dollars equals about Indian 140 rupees. You could get four twelve-ounce bottles of Coke with it, or if you were to eat at a roadside stall, perhaps dish of *daal* (lentils) or vegetables. An entire poor family has to make do with it. If the family earns more than 140 rupees a day, they are deemed to be not poor. Poverty gone, instantaneously.

These are western definitions of poverty in India. Indian figures are even more ridiculous. During the regime of Manmohan Singh, his principal financial adviser was a man called Montek Singh Ahluwalia. Ahluwalia in 2012 set the poverty line at twenty-eight rupees for urban areas and 22.50 rupees for rural areas. That sparked an outrage in India, but it was faux outrage by rich, corrupt politicians living in air-conditioned bungalows in Lutyens' Delhi. The party of Narendra Modi was in the opposition then. They were the biggest decriers of Ahluwalia.

The actual inflation rate in India is estimated at about 10 percent and has been so since 2012, although government estimates are markedly lower. So what do you think Modi has fixed the poverty line at? Thirty-nine rupees for urban areas and thirty-two for rural areas. Accounting for year-on-year inflation, these figures are even more ridiculous than Ahluwalia's. What is the Indian elite thinking? The minimum money that a beggar in India will accept is ten rupees. And the Indian poor are not like America's homeless, or what the latter are deemed to be—addicts and mentally insane and what not. India's poor are a hardworking lot. They are washer men and maids and cycle rickshaw pullers and street hawkers and newspaper deliverymen and every conceivable occupation you can imagine. Often they are up at four a.m. to go to work, and because they are paid by the hour in general, they work until midnight. They live in shabby tenements, eat one meal a deal, wear torn clothes, and often go barefoot. They have no weekends off. Any time lost not doing work is lost earnings.

Donald Trump came to India recently and declared that in a few years, extreme poverty will have disappeared from the face of India, while his friend Modi beamed. Extreme poverty is going nowhere in India. It is only becoming more extreme. It is as extreme as it was in the time of Jehangir or Shah Jehan. The black ghoul of poverty is still very much there in India. The only thing that's changed from the time of Jehangir and Jehan is that the glitterati is larger in number and so is the middle class. But just as the kings and nobles oppressed the poor in Jehangir's time, so too do the rich and the middle class oppress the poor now. And just as they were oblivious to their oppression then, so too are they oblivious to their pain and suffering now.

There is the rural poor in India and then there is the urban poor. Many of the rural poor migrate to the cities for better opportunities, if you can call them that—opportunities to be housemaids and cooks and cleaners and drivers and construction workers of or for the rich and the middle class. In many cases, India is so feudal that the help is seen as being owned by its master or mistress. I will give an example: my first cousin is a rich doctor in Delhi. Her cook's husband has just been murdered. I know the cook and call her regularly, but her mistress, my cousin, is always fretting over who's calling the cook. The cook cannot talk to anyone, even in her free time. Actually, what free time? The cook is like bonded labor, at the disposal of my cousin and her family twenty-four hours a day, seven days a week.

Yelling at the help is very common in India. Actually, many in the privileged classes believe that if you don't yell at the help, it would go out of line. The average Pakistani, because he eats so much more meat, especially beef, than the Indian, is a good head taller. I remember reading a write-up of a famous Indian journalist, Saba Naqvi, who had visited Pakistan. She said that because the help there was so much stronger, employers dare not raise their hands at them, but in India, because the help was much weaker than its Pakistani counterpart, slappings and thrashings of the help abound.

And if the help goes to the police, the police may show some sympathy at first, but once the employer wags some currency notes in the face of the policeman, he will quickly change his tune and start disciplining the help instead.

Life in the city is not easy for the rural migrant. It's almost a similar sort of migration that an Indian student makes to the US. Yes, India didn't afford many great opportunities, but life in the promised land can be tough. The migrant worker immediately faces the twin challenges of shelter and food. Whatever he earns in one day, he consumes that same day itself. Perish the thought of saving money. Migrants rely on human networks from their rural areas who have migrated before to the city—to help find a job, a place to stay, cheap food to eat.

It's a system that seems to work, except that a migrant will most probably end up in a slum, sharing the tenement with any number of people packed chockablock. Talk about social distancing. Sanitation is very poor. Clean drinking water is in short supply. The city sends drinking water trucks but adds tons of chlorine to the water to sanitize it. Many privileged people think that migrants in slums consume a fair share of toddy, so they will not notice the difference when mixing water—clean or chlorinated—into the toddy. Perhaps the best time during the whole day for a migrant is when he's working at a rich person's house, where there is probably an air conditioner on 24-7 and clean water to drink, or when he's asleep in his shanty.

Near my house in a posh neighborhood of Delhi is a vast slum. I have crossed it many times but have never ventured within. Middle-class and rich Indians do not enter slums. There seems to be mud and water and feces and urine everywhere. The whole place stinks to the high heavens. From this paradise, workers emerge to serve the rich and the middle class as cooks and drivers and sweepers. The rich and the middle class do not shake the hands of the poor in India. That was well before the virus came. That will be well after the virus has gone.

Modi insists that the poor are being well fed, but it is clear that he underestimated the impact of the lockdown on them. There are heart-rending images of the poor trying to break through the gates of temples begging for food. Brahmin priests and their relatives live inside the temples, and while they may not be rich, privileged Hindus will make sure that the priests do not go hungry. They will not even go to a safe meeting point to distribute food to the poor, but they will consider it their sacred duty to go to the temple with loads of food and delicacies for the priests. In many cases, they will not touch this food until the priests have eaten first. Modi realized that he erred in underestimating the impact of the lockdown on the poor, but he has stubbornly refused to open more of his treasury. Instead, he has asked the privileged classes to adopt one poor family for food until the crisis ends.

This appeal will of course go nowhere. The rich can take care of their help. The middle class will let go of much of its help, mostly without pay. The compassionate among them will ensure that their furloughed help gets food. Then the question arises where exactly will the privileged classes meet the poor. The rich can send their help to tend to the poor. But the middle classes will have to go themselves to meet the poor. The middle classes are afraid that because the poor lack adequate sanitation, they might pick up the virus from them. That's a fair concern. But the middle class can always leave food at its gate or door (as the case may be) for the poor to pick up themselves.

This arrangement will run into typical self-created Indian confusion. Many middle-class people will argue that the same poor person is going from house to house and collecting more than her fair share of food. Many will wonder that once the pandemic ends, the poor person that they have adopted would keep coming to their door. It's all utter confusion, but it's all self-created. Why not just leave the food outside and fret not over who's picking it up or not? But the Indian brain doesn't work that way. In Hinduism, one can achieve salvation by serving the Brahmins. The Brahmins have been clever with that. They have occupied the top of the caste totem pole and now everybody must serve them.

Whenever there is a birth or a death in a Hindu family, there must be a feast for the Brahmins. Tens if not hundreds of them are gathered and feted with great honor. Recently when I was in India, my old aunt died. There was the customary feast. It is believed that the food one imbibes during the feast reaches the dead person's soul and serves as nourishment for it on its onward journey.

The middle-class Indian is much more comfortable feeding the Brahmins. I can only imagine how much food must be reaching the priests at my neighborhood temple in these pandemic times. The poor of India are mostly from the lower castes. There are many Brahmins who are poor, too, so I must add that it is only the Brahmins who are doubling up as priests and those who are wandering mendicants who are being taken care of by the middle class. The poor Brahmin who isn't overtly spiritual finds herself in the same bucket as the rest of the poor. The poor knew what was going to be their fate. Panic swept the poor in India. They work on a monthly basis in the homes of the rich and the middle class, with no contract whatsoever. If a rich person fires a poor worker during the middle of the month, he retains the rest of the poor man's monthly earnings. Other people are not so callous.

It spread like wildfire that there was a plague in the air. The rich and the middle class started shedding their staff faster than an infected person spreads the coronavirus. The poor knew that they were packed like sardines in their shanties and any sort of social distancing was out of the question for them. They had to rush to their villages. Modi had shut down all vehicular traffic and trains within the country.

In the villages, at least, they would have a mud-hut roof over their heads, more disease distance between them, and a couple of chapatis (breads) to eat per day. But how to reach their villages? Many trekked hundreds of miles from the cities. Many died along the way. In a cruel irony of sorts, when they reached their villages, they were incarcerated. Some were hosed with bleach, as if that would wash the coronavirus away.

Slowly the government came to its senses and started feeding the poor, but it was too little, too late. Modi begged forgiveness from them in a TV address, but many of the poor must not have seen him because they were on the trail home. It was also not clear if their employers would reimburse them their lost wages. Most probably not, because even the rich in India are not feeling that rich right now. And the middle class, just forget it. The middle class says that it has middle-class values, but how those values are being exhibited during this pandemic in India beats me. The economy in India was already on the skids before the virus struck, and now that it is practically destroyed, it will be a while before people start feeling and acting generous.

The exodus of the poor in India is a great tragedy. Modi should have planned for it. Instead he went for a full-bore instant lockdown.

Whenever the lockdown ends, the task will be to revive the economy. If Modi can do that, everything will be forgotten, for Indians, especially the poor, are a forgiving people. If the economy languishes, then Modi is toast. For Gandhi made sure that he gave the poor, man and woman, an ultimate weapon against the vagaries of the privileged classes, and that was the vote. Six to eight hundred million people can determine the political fate of a nation of 1.4 billion. Modi knows that. Every politician in India knows that. Knowing that is the only reason why there is still somewhat of a check on the greed and the callousness of India's privileged classes, a greed and a callousness that you have to see to believe. That's why they are kept in somewhat in check from their depredations against the poor. Until the poor have the vote, and the ability to decide the fate of governments, there will not be a revolution in India. Amen.

CHAPTER SIX

JUGAAD (INDIGENOUS INGENUITY)

Jugaad is a term for Indian ingenuity, never more necessary than it is now. With a lockdown in place, the financial ministry in New Delhi found itself with an unusual problem: the amended finance bill passed by Parliament could not be printed on government presses without obtaining written orders in physical form. Enter jugaad—Indian ingenuity. A demi-official letter was generated under a rule change that carried the phone number of the signatory. The number was then called, and the finance bill was printed in plenty of time. This sort of figuring out solutions on the fly is occurring throughout the government, including having "fully sanitized" messengers sent to officials whenever signed documents are necessary.

But what about jugaad and the increasing rate of hunger in India? During this pandemic India's working poor have become India's begging poor, with migrant workers stranded far from their villages and dependent on handouts with no work in sight.

The increasing numbers of those going hungry due to being stranded and out of work after the lockdown must be fed. Any proposed solution needs to incorporate a balanced strategy using proven initiatives in innovative ways. This is jugaad.

China built two hospitals with a capacity of twenty-six hundred beds in just over a week. "China has a record of getting things done fast even for monumental projects like this," says Yanzhong Huang, a senior fellow for global health at the Council on Foreign Relations. "This authoritarian country relies on this top-down mobilization approach. They can overcome bureaucratic nature and financial constraints and are able to mobilize all of the resources," he points out.

As the pandemic hit, America did not have enough hospital beds for COVID patients. America knew that it could not emulate China and magically create hospital beds out of nothing. The US Army Corps of Engineers was summoned. They identified the Javits Convention Center in New York City and converted it into a two-thousand-bed hospital in record time. They have also converted the McCormick Place Convention Center in Chicago into a three-thousand-bed hospital. The army is nothing if not authoritarian. Perhaps only authoritarian entities can do such magical things.

The navy has two ships that are dedicated hospitals. Yes, of course. If you send your fleet to China and there are large casualties, what better way to treat them than to have hospitals at hand? Or at sea, to be more accurate. The US has two hospital ships, the USNS *Mercy* and the USNS *Comfort*, each with a capacity of one thousand beds. They are nearly three American football fields long and ten stories high, making them indisputably the largest hospital ships in the world.

The ships are so massive, each would be tantamount to the fourth-biggest hospital in the United States. Imagine that, in a country dotted with large hospitals. The USNS *Mercy* and USNS *Comfort* are equipped with twelve operating rooms, a blood bank, a medical laboratory, a pharmacy, an optometry lab, and a CT scanner. I guess if you want to rule the world, you've got to rule the world like this. The *Comfort* was dispatched off the coast of New York and the *Mercy* (May the good Lord have mercy upon us!) off the coast of California. They could be redeployed to other hot spots like, say, New Orleans.

India has almost as long a coastline as its land borders. It is a peninsula, after all. On the west is eternal enemy Pakistan. On the east lurks another enemy, China. India can take care of Pakistan in a jiffy. It's like that math course that you know you are going to ace, so you love prepping for it. India is obsessed with Pakistan. But anyone who's obsessed with a rat cannot be a greater than a cat. China is building a fearsome navy, with aircraft carriers and whatnot. India aims to build a blue-water navy, but it struggles. It imports an aircraft carrier from Russia, but it takes years to arrive in India because it has to be rejigged and retrofitted. India does not even have a hospital ship.

So no ability to build hospitals in real time, no ability to convert vast convention centers into instant hospitals, no floating hospital ships. What was Modi going to do? He hit upon a typical jugaadi (indigenous ingenuity) brain wave. In Gujarat, he had placed solar panels over farmlands. Now he would convert his trains into hospitals.

It is important to know that Modi had suspended service of the vast railway passenger network. It was the first time in the history of the Indian railways that passenger service was suspended. Passenger service started in India in 1853. This was the first time in 167 years of rail service in India that passenger service had been suspended. Imagine that! India fought a short but brutal war with China in 1962, a similarly short but brutal engagement with Pakistan in 1948, and two fairly long engagements with Pakistan in 1965 and 1971. Freight trains are a prime target in war for the enemy from the air, because they carry matériel. Passenger trains, too, because they carry men—that is, soldiers. In any case, from twenty thousand feet up, it is hard to distinguish a freight train from a passenger train. All trains look the same. But India did not suspend its passenger train service even during wartime. Eight billion passengers take the rail in India every year. All of these passengers, or a subset of these, let's say half, four billion stranded. Left high and dry. No road service, either.

Modi is flying blind with almost no testing. Still if you return from overseas, you get mandatorily tested, and if you have clear COVID symptoms, they do test you. Per capita, India has fewer hospital beds and ventilators than almost any country in the world. India has 2.3 intensive care beds per hundred thousand people. By contrast, China has 3.6 and the United States nearly 35 per hundred thousand people.

As for ventilators, the government doesn't publish numbers. But experts quoted in Indian media estimate that there are between thirty and forty thousand ventilators nationwide. Even with its vastly superior medical facilities, the coronavirus has wreaked havoc in the US. Imagine the havoc it could wrought in India. Modi had to do something. In a desperate display of jugaad, he ordered that trains be converted into standing hospitals.

About 20,000twenty thousand train compartments have been converted into isolation wards for coronavirus patients. Indian Railways runs 125 hospitals across the nation, so it already has the expertise to expand into medical service. According to Indian Railways, mosquito nets and charging points for mobile phones and laptops have been fitted in the compartments, and space has been created for paramedics. The network is also considering hiring more doctors or reemploying retired medical staff.

Good on you, Modi. Now you have to get a bit more systematic and less jugaadi. Order your private sector to build more ventilators. Some folks, like the Mahindra Group, are already doing so. And even though your COVID cases are few for now, start building temporary hospitals in places like cricket stadiums. You took Donald Trump to see the world's largest cricket stadium, a spanking-new one built in Motera in the state of Gujarat. There Trump addressed 125,000 with his customary élan or demagoguery—take your pick. Well, that stadium and so many others dotted far and wide across your vast land will make for ideal makeshift hospitals. And creating these hospitals will generate employment. You might have to tear them apart later, but at least you are paying people for doing work rather than sitting idle.

The tempest is coming, Modi. Get ready for it. You are seen as a man of action. Make it happen.

CHAPTER SEVEN

COUNTRY
OF LIGHTS

Vishnu, Shiva, and Brahma constitute Hinduism's holy trinity. Vishnu is the
preserver of the world, Shiva the destroyer, and Brahma the creator. Brahma
is not worshipped for reasons beyond the scope of this text. Shiva is fiercely
worshipped, and Vishnu is worshipped mainly in the form of his two avatars
on earth: the seventh avatar, Rama, and the eighth avatar, Krishna. Westerners will be familiar with the Hare Rama Hare Krishna movement.

Ram's life is chronicled in the Hindu epic the Ramayana. Ram is a
model of rectitude, his life one of extreme sacrifice. If you are a Hindu and
you read the Ramayana, you will start crying, as I did. So good is Ram, so
deep the injustice meted out to him. Ram is banished to the forest for
fourteen long years along with his wife and younger brother. His wife gets
kidnapped; he rescues her and returns triumphantly to his home city of
Ayodhya to reclaim his kingdom. Hindus celebrate that day as the festival
of lights. They light their homes and businesses with *diyas* (earthen lamps)
and candles.

Hindus pray to many gods and goddesses. One of them is Lakshmi,
who is actually Vishnu's consort, and who is seen as the goddess of wealth
and prosperity. But what good is Lakshmi if she cannot enter your doors?
So Hindus fling open their doors on the occasion of Diwali. And since
the goddess won't enter a dirty home, all homes are painted and polished
and cleaned well before Diwali. It is a Hindu trait to keep one's home

spick-and-span; it's just the neighborhood that she doesn't care about, flinging her trash and garbage by the road. In the mid-nineties, a plague hit Delhi, which frightened everyone enough so that they became more careful, but then people have returned to type. In any case, why discuss dirt during the happy occasion of Diwali?

A worship is typically held, sweetmeats and food are partaken of in plenty, and then many people gather with their friends and family to gamble the night away. Crackers start bursting days before Diwali and, on Diwali night proper, reach a crescendo. It's as if the heavens have burst. Smoke fills the air. In India's heavily polluted cities like Delhi and Mumbai, further pollution is crammed in. But people don't care. Everyone is out to outdo their neighbor with fancier and bigger crackers. Crackers, lit with a match, bundles of crackling joy—and air pollution.

With the intense pollution of Indian cities, crackers are slowly going out fashion. State governments are banning them during Diwali. But that is like banning turkey during Thanksgiving. Crackers are a once-a-year event. Pollution is year-round. Much of India's glitterati and the rich applaud the ban on crackers because they want to live in a clean India, but the middle class is nostalgic for the fun of old. So much about India is changing. Ironically, the lockdown, having cleared the streets of traffic, is clearing the air.

Midway through the lockdown, India's chatterati were getting restless. There had hardly been a hundred COVID deaths. In a country of 1.3 billion, that amounted to virtually nothing. Indians easily slaughter over ten times that number of people during an intercommunal riot. Modi had gone too far, felt many Indians. Much of India was vegetarian, and even those who ate meat made sure to consume enough vegetables. Many Indians subscribe to the view that vegetables come out of the ground and are thus naturally safer than animals, for who knows what they ate. An Indian restaurateur in Beijing told me that a Chinese man joked with him that the Chinese eat anything that moves and the Indian anything that grows. That's exactly what many Indians think. This coronavirus is for the bat-eating and rat-eating Chinese or the beef-eating Westerner, but why us? Even if we eat meat, it's just chicken and mutton (goat meat). Many

Indians were convinced that Modi had fired the starter's pistol too fast on the lockdown.

The chatterati have enormous influence, dominating the TV waves and the internet. The way they vote, that's who gets elected. Modi is their darling. In many countries with the extreme and almost inerasable poverty of India's, there might have been a revolution. But not so in India. Hindus are a fatalistic lot, and the Hindu poor extremely so. They feel that if misery was their lot in this lifetime, they just have to grin and bear it. The next lifetime might turn out better.

Modi has a pulse on the middle class. He sensed that they were, in a manner of speaking, going mad. But he knew he was on the right track in the fight against COVID-19. He wasn't going to lift the lockdown anytime soon. Then he had a brainstorm. Or maybe it was someone else's brainstorm that he made his own.

On April 6, Modi ordered his countrymen and women to shut off all electric lights in their homes and come outside and light diyas and candles. Those who could not light diyas could shine their mobile phones toward the sky. Many Hindus light a diya or two in their house every day. They found no reason not to comply with Modi's diktat.

On April 6 at nine p.m. Indian Standard Time, a strange sight was seen at the International Space Station. The Indian subcontinent, otherwise brightly lit, went completely off the map. Slowly but surely, it was a replaced by a warm, diffused glow. It was as if all of the subcontinent had merged into one. It seemed that there wasn't any harshness of bright lights anywhere. It was as if the soul of India had become one. Modi the master had achieved his aim. He had tapped into the religious sentiments of Indians to achieve his aims.

LIGHT, RELIGION, CRICKET—THE VIRUS DOESN'T CARE.

But isn't Modi supposed to be the secular leader of a secular nation? What would India's Muslims think, for instance? To the Hindus, their diyas, to the Christians, their candles, but Muslims didn't believe in diyas and were not so big on candles, so would they be the ones who would be shining their cell phones as torches? Like everything else in India, the lockdown too has become communalized. I live in the Nizamuddin East area of Delhi. Across the road is a Muslim ghetto. I have been in it only once, but seeing the carcasses of cows hanging from hooks, I almost threw up. I was young then, in my late teens. When I was even younger, my classmate was a Muslim girl called Sabiha Hassan Sultana. She trusted me and would ask me to accompany her to her bus stop located next to the ghetto.

Inside the ghetto is a shrine to an Indian Muslim saint, Nizamuddin Auliya. He lived from 1238 to 1325 AD. You can imagine how old Islam is in India. Nizamuddin was a Sufi saint, albeit Sunni, who preached moderation.

One extreme offshoot of Islam in India has been a movement called the Tablighi Jamaat, which mandates that Islam should be practiced the way it was during the time of the prophet of Islam. Followers of Tablighi Jamaat feel that many deviancies have entered Islam—for instance, they abhor a moderate form of Islam called Sufism. They are Sunni to the core and do not even regard the Shias as Muslim. Saint Nizamuddin would not have brooked them.

Ironically a big meeting of Tablighis was organized near the shrine of Nizamuddin in early March. About nine thousand people from all parts of India and overseas attended the event. The Delhi police had issued rulings against large gatherings, but the police tend to ignore religious violations, because any enforcement can lead to a communal riot. By April 18, 4,291 confirmed cases of COVID-19 in India, about a third of all, had been linked to this gathering. Hundreds have died owing to the infection from the meeting. Indian officials have estimated that more than a third of the country's cases were connected to Tablighi Jamaat, which held a huge gathering of preachers in India in March. Similar meetings in Malaysia and Pakistan have also led to outbreaks.

The government was then forced to race to track down any and all congregants and quarantine them all. Masked police have since sealed off the headquarters on all sides and are policing the area with assault rifles. One Muslim man who was allowed under lockdown to keep his milk stall open to sell milk to everyone said, "Fear is staring at us, from everywhere."

Because of mounting blame being heaped on Muslims, he said, "People need only a small reason to beat us or lynch us." But it is the density of the crowd that matters. The virus loves people in close quarters. The virus could care less if the crowd has congregated for a religious gathering or a cricket match.

As of this writing, in many villages Muslim traders are barred from entering because of their faith. But it isn't the name of the religion that is to blame, but the size of the crowd. The seventy-year-old Sikh preacher Baldev Singh had returned from a trip to Europe's virus epicenter, Italy (and Germany), before he went preaching in more than a dozen villages in Punjab. Singh and his two associates, who tested positive for the virus along with Singh, ignored orders to self-isolate once they were home in India and continued on with their preaching tour until Singh died of the virus.

India was stunned. A popular Punjabi singer who lives in Canada, Sidhu Moose Wala, released a song about the virus that was viewed 2.3 million times on YouTube in less than two days. The song is about Baldev Singh's fatal pilgrimage and includes the lyric "I passed on the disease . . . roaming around the village like a shadow of death." Punjab's police chief is now encouraging residents to listen to the song as a warning.

The lockdown in India has been fierce, somewhat like the lockdown in Wuhan, China, and quite unlike the shelter in place in the US. In India, hardly any restaurant is open for takeout. Pizza and other food can be delivered, but a pizza delivery man tested positive a few days ago, further hitting sales of the food delivery business. People are allowed to go outside to walk in the States. Not so in India. Flights are not flying, and trains and buses are not running. If you step out, a cop hauls you over and asks where you are headed. All private and government businesses are shuttered.

Countries that have done a good job so far containing the spread of the virus have refrained from imposing a complete nationwide lockdown. These include Singapore, Taiwan, and Germany. Even China placed only Hubei Province, which includes Wuhan, under complete lockdown.

State governors such as Arvind Kejriwal of Delhi and Mamata Banerjee of West Bengal, who typically are inveterate critics of Modi, now talk respectfully about him. Kejriwal addresses Modi as "sir" now. You don't see state governors like Andrew Cuomo of New York or Gretchen Whitmer of Michigan giving extended daily press briefings and seemingly preening to become president or vice president.

Modi is seen as a tough enforcer of laws. With his light-a-lamp crusade, he also emerged as the nation's healer in chief. All of India is praying with Modi. With diyas and candles.

CHAPTER EIGHT

TREAT ME, DOC, OR I WILL TREAT YOU

After independence in 1947, the two main occupations open to an Indian man were the military or the civil services. By the sixties and the seventies, India was producing large numbers of doctors and engineers. Many of these doctors started migrating to the West, notably the US and the UK. It seemed that Indian doctors had taken over the National Health Service in the UK. As when anything colored becomes popular in a white country, there was a backlash. The American government swiftly stopped administering the United States Medical Licensing Examination in India.

India, in the seventies and eighties and even nineties, was under a cloud of socialism. In fact, it was a cloudy sort of socialism, for on the one side there was the vast government and public sector, and on the other a small private sector. Economic reforms unleashed in 1991 not only dismantled the public sector but they also fostered a wave of entrepreneurship in the country. Many people, unshackled by regulations and laws—the infamous license, permit, quota raj as it was then called—started making a lot of money. The United States Medical Licensing Examination was administered in places like Bangkok and Singapore. Many Indians could now afford to go to these faraway places and take the exam.

By 2015, doctors could make the big bucks in India. Except that they could make five times bigger bucks in the States. The stories people would relate about Indian doctors in the States—McMansions, luxury cars and many of them, untold wealth and respect. But doctors in India could get respect, too. It took a crisis like COVID to figure out if that was true.

COVID struck Italy, then the US, hard. The clanging of bells and utensils to show solidarity with medical professionals began to be a nightly rallying cry. Not so in India. Indian doctors and nurses were thrown out of their houses by their neighbors for fear that they were carrying the infection. They couldn't sleep in their homes at night. These very neighbors, were they to fall sick, would be begging these very same doctors and nurses to save their lives. Modi appeared on TV and begged people to back off. They didn't take heed, even to their messiah. Life came first to them, then devotion. And Modi was only a man, not god. Callous a response as this was, it was no more callous than Modi's neglecting to put transportation options in place when he moved to shut down the country in a mere four hours.

Delhi's state governor got into the act and reserved rooms in one of Delhi's best hotels, the Lalit, for the medical staff. It must have been the most sensible, the most noble thing he has ever done. Ratan Tata, one of India's foremost industrialists, runs a network of some of the world's finest hotels across India. He opened all his hotels to medical professionals.

But worse was in store for medical personnel. They were undergoing contact tracing of the aforementioned Tablighi Jamaat in one of Delhi's Muslim neighborhoods when suddenly rocks and stones started raining on them. They were risking their lives to identify people with COVID infections and save the lives of locals. Instead, the locals were coming after their lives. The head of the Tablighi Jamaat in India went missing for weeks until he was finally apprehended.

No wonder Indian doctors and nurses want to leave for the States. The money is much better, the treatment much better. Doctors and nurses in India are meant to treat; instead, very often they get the treatment. Did I also tell you that Indian doctors in India know that doctors in the States are revered? The image of the American god-doc has been etched in my mind since I read Arthur Hailey's *Strong Medicine*. In this time of crisis in the States, the country is relaxing rules for foreign doctors to get in. Many more of India's doctors and nurses will surely be making a beeline for the States.

Doctors and nurses are not the only ones receiving the brunt of India's panicked rage.

Indian people with East Asian features comprise about fifteen to twenty million people, mostly concentrated in the country's northeast. Many such people have moved to Delhi for greener pastures, where they are often derogatorily called *chink*. Their women are fairer than the average Indian woman, so are in heavy demand for sex by men of the plains, but when it comes to marriage, they disdain them for their eyes. They have never really integrated into Indian society. If you go to their homelands, they will often ask you if you have come from India. They don't consider themselves a part of India. "If you don't accept me, how can I accept you," goes their logic.

Due to the supposedly Chinese origins of the virus, many of these Indians, especially those living in the plains, have had to bear racial slurs.

The most testing for coronavirus that India is doing today is of people returning from overseas or of people displaying obvious symptoms of the virus. That is why the number of active cases is so low. There is no large-scale testing of people within the country. When a person enters the country, he or she is forced to go under a fourteen-day quarantine. If they quarantine themselves in a house, the local police mark that house with an X sign and put up an accompanying notice.

Indians are nosy by nature. Neighbors take pictures of the X sign and the police notice and circulate them along with the quarantined person's address throughout the neighborhood. Then that house is treated as if the bubonic plague had set on it. How utterly pitiless!

A crisis can bring out the best in people. It can also bring out the worst. It is sad that COVID-19 is showing the ugly underbelly of some of India's chatterati. As for India's doctors and nurses making a beeline for the States, they will be much more welcome in their adopted land.

CHAPTER NINE

AFTER THE LOCKDOWN

Modi's repeated plea to the nation was that India did not have nearly the sophisticated medical systems of Italy and America (though many Americans will beg to disagree with that assertion), and that he must flatten the peak so as not to overwhelm India's health-care system.

In India "social distancing" is more often referred to as "disease distancing." India is a very touchy-feely culture. Full-throated hugs between men have always been common. Now American-style hugs between men and women as well as women and women have become common as well. So has the kiss on the cheek, especially among the elites. This too is copycat American culture.

Men and boys readily hold hands. When I first came to Purdue University at age twenty-one to do my PhD, my roommates and I were holding hands in public until some Americans laughed at us. Women too in India have held hands since time immemorial. There is nothing homosexual about men holding hands or women holding hands. It is completely to show amity. Men and women holding hands in public is a recent phenomenon and is a direct result of the impact of American culture. When a man holds a woman's hands, especially if they are of the same culture, then that in general signifies that they are a couple. Still, a sister might cling to her brother's arm, and there is nothing amorous about that.

Untouchability is not practiced much in cities and towns with their crowded public infrastructure like buses, trains, and metros. The practice of untouchability is more common in villages. In cities and towns, the domestic help, even frequently the cook (the kitchen is considered almost sacrosanct in Indian culture) can be from the untouchable class. Many Indians will not inquire the caste of the person they hire as the help.

With Muslims, eating together outside in restaurants is passé. Where many Hindus have a problem is eating in Muslim homes. They feel that the utensils are contaminated by the Muslims eating beef, the cow, of course, being sacred to many Hindus. But Hindus will not have a problem eating at the houses of Westerners, especially whites, even though they are well aware that the Westerner could be eating beef as well.

At parties, it is very common for men to put their arms around one another or tap one another on the knee or thigh or even keep your hand on the knee and thigh of another man for prolonged periods. It's just male bonding. Indians love to touch and feel. Touching the feet of the elderly is de rigueur. Even with foreign friends sometimes, for instance the French, I start touching their legs when seated on a sofa, and I am immediately and constantly reprimanded. I feel like a fool, and ensure that my hands don't go roaming off again.

Modi's drastic decision to impose his lockdown early seems to be working. But there is a key issue. India is testing very little. The US has done twelve thousand tests per one million of its population, Italy twenty-three thousand. India has done a paltry three hundred per million. Without testing, Modi is flying blind. If he had tested much more, he would have discovered many more cases and could have isolated them.

It is very unlikely that Modi will be able to extend his lockdown much longer. The Indian economy was already on the skids before the virus arrived. Now it might even contract. It could take years for the economy to recover. Modi will certainly open the country gradually. But open it he must. He has played all his cards. Now his country is broke and, according to David Beasley, executive director of the World Food Programme, on the verge of a hunger pandemic.

Social distancing helps flatten the curve, prevent spikes, and reduce the number of infected cases. But it also prevents something called herd immunity. Herd immunity is when a large section of the population develops immunity against the disease, if contracted either asymptomatically or symptomatically. In the latter case, the patient has, of course, to live to tell the tale. Herd immunity can also develop from a vaccine, which seems far away, although researchers at Oxford University are confident that they will have one out by September. All power to them.

Sweden is trying the concept of herd immunity and failing. It has close to two thousand deaths. Its Scandinavian neighbors, like Denmark, Norway, and Finland, are all practicing some form of lockdown or the other. Denmark has close to four hundred deaths, Norway close to two hundred, and Finland about 150. Clearly Sweden is failing, but it is intransigent on herd immunity. Herd immunity is a questionable premise; COVID-19 is so new no one knows how many antibodies develop in an infected person and how much immunity she gets. Many scientists propagating herd immunity are just basing their argument upon how the body reacts to conventional virus. COVID-19 seems to mutate quite fast, making it difficult to even develop a vaccine against it.

People in the United States are fed up, even with a lockdown more limited in scope than India's. But then America is the land of the free and the home of the brave, and Trump was elected on a campaign of majoritarian discontent. People want the freedom they feel their vote for Trump guaranteed.

Modi was also elected on a majoritarian campaign. India's Hindus consider him their pied piper. Before the virus arrived, Modi was flailing. He had in fact put the Indian state of Kashmir under lockdown for months, stripping Kashmir of its statehood in an effort to "bring prosperity and equality to the area." In a lockdown much more stringent than the one he imposed on India on March 24, in Kashmir, even the internet and mobile phone services were banned. Modi had become a master at imposing lockdowns. But not in reopening them. Kashmir will probably not open up when the rest of India opens up in May.

Modi was flailing also because he had offered minorities in several neighboring countries refuge in India. He said that these minorities—Hindu, Christian, Buddhist, Jain, Sikh, and Parsi—were heavily persecuted in Pakistan, Bangladesh, and Afghanistan. But Shia Muslims and Muslim Ahmaddiyas are also heavily persecuted in Pakistan. One of the most persecuted communities in the world is the Muslim Rohingya community in Myanmar. Modi's scheme had no place for Muslims. And frankly it seems to have had a place for Christians only to mute voices in the West.

Muslims in India rebelled against Modi's discriminatory policies. Many liberal Hindus joined. There were horrific riots in Delhi between Muslims and conservative Hindus on the day that Donald Trump was visiting Delhi, just eleven miles from where he was. It was India's day of shame. The emperor of the world is visiting your home, and you are busy killing one another.

Modi was ashamed. He was losing popularity. But conservative Hindus are his base, just as orthodox Christians are Trump's. Modi took only perfunctory action against the rioters. He could not punish the Hindus, so he had to let go of the Muslims as well. While firmly ensconced in power, Modi realized that his government was going nowhere. The virus seems to have come at the right time for Modi to show what a decisive leader he is.

First the advisory in the US by Dr. Anthony Fauci and other medical professionals such as Dr. Sanjay Gupta was against wearing masks. They claimed that the virus was so minute it would go through a cloth mask. Then a month or so later, they said that there were not enough simple masks around for medical professionals. Now the advisory is to wear a mask.

The trouble with the US is that it has lost its manufacturing. Making masks became such a tough task. An acclaimed designer came on TV and showed that he was making the simplest possible cloth masks, one with a metal rim for the nose. He said the biggest challenge was inserting a metal rim. Asked about how many masks his crew was making per day, he said a hundred. Then I saw a machine, made in China, of course, that was churning out a hundred masks in minutes.

Indians are wearing masks of all kinds, and in Delhi an Indian can receive a sentence of six months in jail for not wearing a mask. Clearly, while the lockdown may slowly be lifted, there will be changes in how Indians live that will endure.

Just like things get politicized in the US, they get communalized in India. Right-wing Hindu hate-mongers are accusing the Muslim Tablighi Jamaat of being a super-spreader of the virus. Sure, the Jamaat did a very wrong thing in holding a very large gathering in Delhi. But so did the ruling BJP (Modi's party, a Hindu faith–based organization) governor of the large Indian state of Uttar Pradesh, a Hindu holy monk called Yogi Adityanath, hold a large gathering without enforcing social distance in the Hindu temple town of Ayodhya. It was just fortunate that the virus didn't spread from there and instead spread from the Jamaat.

Hindu right-wingers are resorting to their favorite pastime of bashing Muslims and labeling the coronavirus the Tablighi virus. The virus is no more the Tablighi virus than it is the Chinese virus or the Wuhan virus. These defamatory wounds will take a long time to heal in India. Fortunately there are powerful state governors like Uddhav Thackeray of Maharashtra, Arvind Kejriwal of Delhi, and Mamata Banerjee of West Bengal who are fighting against the menace of communalism. Any one of them could become India's prime minister one day.

And what about Modi? He lamely tweeted that the virus does not see any religion, but he hasn't gone on TV to assert the fact. Modi cannot cut himself away from his right-wing hate-mongering Hindu base, for they are his trusted vote bank. The purpose of this writing is not to absolve the Jamaat for what they did. The willful disregard of authority that they exhibited was entirely careless and downright dangerous, but they didn't know that they would become a super-spreader. Yogi Adityanath could have become a super-spreader. What would the Hindu right wing have done then? Beat up on one of their own? Impossible.

India is a beautiful secular country. India's Constitution follows the doctrine of separation of church from state. Modi and other leaders of India must ensure this doctrine. By this doctrine, a Yogi Adityanath should not even be in power. We have seen that wherever this doctrine has been flouted, like, say, in Islamic countries, they have mostly gone to seed. The

West has followed this doctrine more or less diligently, until of course demagogues like Trump came along.

The task for Modi after he lifts the lockdown is to scale up testing. But efforts in that regard are proving lackluster in India. If testing doesn't happen on a large scale, he will not know who has the virus and who doesn't and whom to quarantine and whom not to. As social distancing norms are relaxed, a very large proportion of the population could be asymptomatic carriers of the virus. The US failed in testing, and look where it has found itself. Testing is absolutely fundamental to stem the rot of the virus in India. India has extinguished two pandemics—smallpox and polio—with a very concerted effort. I have been involved with the Rotary organization, and I know that Rotary played a very active role in eradicating polio. Perhaps Rotary or Lions or a similar India-wide organization can be roped in to tackle COVID as well.

Like Trump, Modi has to get his economy on track. But as he eases the lockdown, and if there is a spike in cases, what will he do?

If there is a severe spike in cases, he might have to go recidivist and impose another lockdown. That would be devastating for the economy, as well as for people's psyche. Right now, the best-case scenario for Modi is that God has chosen Indians as his own people, and that the virus has not spread widely in the country. But again we are down to testing. India has imported about six hundred thousand rapid test kits from China, but these have proven to be faulty. Abbott Laboratories in the US appears to have developed a reliable rapid test kit, but with the need in the US intense, it is unclear if it can spare any for India.

For sure, most Indians will wear masks as they return to their offices and factories after the lockdown. For sure, many will practice social distancing as much as possible. People in India are using videoconferencing facilities like Zoom, but apparently it has a security defect, so Google has banned its use. The Indian government has also now banned its use, although the country's defense minister and the senior-most minister in the cabinet, Rajnath Singh, was seen blissfully using Zoom recently. The Indian government has offered close to half a million dollars (in purchasing power terms) to any Indian who can come up with an alternative to Zoom.

That again is a tall ask, for Indians have not been very prolific in coming up with their apps that can work at scale.

Unlike many Americans, who live alone, Indians live together in crowded apartments. If a person is single, she might go for an Airbnb-type arrangement in a city, also known as paying guest. Depending upon the arrangement, she will interact with her host family. Families tend to live together, with often three or even four generations under one roof. Offices, too, are crowded. Only the top staff has any office, with most of the subordinates confined to booths. One industry that is getting badly hurt by the virus is the offshoring industry in India. With poor broadband facilities at home and cramped quarters, it is virtually impossible to work from home. Many Western firms offshoring to India are changing their plans. Many are using artificial intelligence to eliminate the need for humans. Australia's Telstra and Britain's Virgin Media, both of whom have offshore units in India, have announced plans to recruit hundreds of people back home.

Many experts are predicting that the virus will return in full force in the Northern Hemisphere once the winter months begin. This would be catastrophic for the world. The United States has done four million tests, just above 1 percent of its population. India has done four hundred thousand tests. India seems to be in testing where the US was a couple months ago—flailing. But the US seems to be getting its act together. India barely so. I predict that if a second wave hits India this winter, it be as behind the testing curve as the US found itself and will be caught as unawares as the US when the first wave hit it.

A vaccine seems to be the panacea. But Indian generic pharmaceutical companies are not known for their innovation. They are trying, but it seems likely that a vaccine will emerge from somewhere else. An Indian firm might get the license to produce the vaccine en masse, something that is their forte. But a vaccine seems far off, a year or two away, no matter what the researchers at Oxford claim.

There is a theory that if there is a second wave of the virus, then a lockdown could mitigate its effects, and slowly but surely, one could strangulate the virus until the vaccine arrives. But this theory is unfounded in fact. Lifting the lockdown now could result in a heavy spike, even when summer is impending. There is no proof of any herd mentality. Sweden's experiment in this regard has proven disastrous, to say the least. In the winter months, the virus could emerge as a hydra-headed monster. So, another lockdown. But once the lockdown lifts, out comes the virus in full force. The world, including India, might have to live with the virus until a vaccine arrives.

Americans and Indians are similar in that they are prudes. They are not like the French at all, for whom sex is part of life and something beautiful. Americans indulge in sex and talk about it a little. Indians pretend that they do not indulge in sex and never talk about it. But the stork is not bringing all the new babies to India. Attraction between sexes is one great impediment to working from home. Now with kids at home all the time, Indian couples are finding it even more difficult to find moments for intimacy. But the desire for sex remains strong, just as the thirst for freedom and stupidity runs deep in the heart of that idiotic man in Kentucky brandishing his AK-47 in public. The first time I saw the man in Kentucky waving the AK-47, I thought he was a military man. Then I saw so many others. I have never seen so many assault rifles in my life. I didn't even know you could buy an AK-47 in the States. Gun control, what's that, eh?

Let's revert to sex. The *New York Times* is full about articles about the pandemic, but I have seen only one article in it about sex and the virus. In Indian media, just forget it. It is well established that the virus sheds from the nose, mouth, and rectum, all orifices used in the sex act. Right now with families confined to their own homes, there is a danger, but a small danger, of someone contracting the virus from an asymptomatic person. What happens when the lockdown lifts? Each family member will go their own way—to schools and colleges and offices and factories. There they will perforce come in contact with many more people than they are during the lockdown, and often in close contact.

What if a woman returns home with the virus? She is asymptomatic and she hasn't been tested. She continues her romantic relations with her partner. Sex is a very powerful force, and once in the act, people might be tempted to drop all inhibitions, virus be damned. Sex is also the most primordial of forces, so not easily repudiated at all. Now you have two people infected at home. It may not be long before the kids get infected. More than 70 percent of the population in India is above fifteen. Let's assume that 60 percent is above eighteen. That means over eight hundred million people could be sexually active. Divide eight hundred million by half, and you get four hundred million men and four hundred million women. All of this eight hundred million could spread the virus. Then with the lockdown over, neighbors drop by one neighbor's for a cup of tea. They sit together on a sofa and then transmit the virus that way.

All of this may sound like hyperbole, but the panic that has gripped the US and many countries in Europe hasn't hit India as yet. That is because a death count of six hundred is nothing in a country of 1.4 billion. In any case, life is valued less in India than in the West. It is only when the death count goes to hundreds of thousands, even a million, that India will truly wake up to the need for testing. It's a horrendous thought, the death count, but it may come true. Unless God shines his light on India.

CHAPTER TEN

PHILANTHROPY INDIAN STYLE AND WHAT WILL HAPPEN NEXT

Many questions loom. First and foremost, what does the future hold for the virus in India, and secondly, has the lockdown done any good? The answers are evolving every day. As of this writing, India has tested fewer than one hundred thousand people in total, which is approximately 694 tests per million people. This is one of the lowest rates in the world, and the number of tests per million varies widely from state to state. An increase in testing is necessary to reach a level of transparency regarding accurate answers. As for the lockdown, the word of mouth among epidemiologists and other health care experts is that you don't know where you are with the virus today. You only always know where you were two weeks ago. To put it mildly, then, the jury's out.

But one thing is certain—in this time of worldwide crisis, India's rich and superrich have lagged behind the rest of the world in how much they give back to the country in which they made their wealth. For instance, none of the dollar millionaires or billionaires offered shelter or transportation home to the stranded migrant workers, a simple and generous thing to do. Many of these billionaires do contribute to religious institutions, which is not considered philanthropy. But the generosity of reaching out with financial relief to the actual poor has been sorely lacking.

According to the OECD, the pretax share of the national income of the top 1 percent in India was a whopping 22 percent in 2017. India is a $3 trillion economy. Domestic philanthropic funding was close $1.8 billion between 2013 and 2017, again according to the OECD. International philanthropy for India was $1.2 billion for the years 2013 to 2015. Assume a constant distribution over the years, domestic philanthropy stands at $0.36 billion a year, while international philanthropy is $0.4 billion a year.

Domestic philanthropy has started to match international philanthropy. But giving by Indian philanthropists and corporate bodies, especially the top 1 percent, is paltry compared to what they are earning and compared to the percentages in the rest of the world.

One man, Azim Premji, son of the founder of Western Indian Vegetable Products, took over, abbreviated the name of the company to Wipro, and transformed this manufacturer of cooking oil into a global information technology company, known for its commitment to sustainability and good corporate citizenship. Premji has pledged that 80 percent of his wealth will go to charity through his foundation. Such a high level of charity is rare in India. A friend who used to work at Wipro said that Premji was giving all this money to his foundation to avoid taxes, but be that as it may, Premji seems like an extremely generous man. With a giving total of approximately $21 billion, Azim Premji is now in the top ranks of givers, along with Bill and Melinda Gates and Warren Buffett.

It is clear the rich in India hold their bills close to their chest. Partly, this is due to the newness of such extreme wealth to these individuals. Sure, there are the Tatas and the Birlas and the Bajajs and the Sarabhais, industrialists and merchants who made their wealth before independence, but let's consider India's richest and Asia's second-richest billionaire, Mukesh Ambani, who is worth north of $40 billion. His father, Dhirubhai Ambani, created his empire in the seventies and eighties, and Mukesh has taken the empire to new heights. The Tatas and the Birlas have been

renowned in India for their philanthropy since time immemorial. Ambani
is not. His wife runs a school for the children of the rich set in Mumbai.
That's mostly what is known about Mukesh's charity.

Before economic reforms were unleashed in 1991, India did not have a
single dollar billionaire (in real exchange terms). Since then the country
has spouted 131. In terms of dollar billionaires, India now just ranks
behind the US (585) and China (476). This is an enormous development.
Most of these billionaires are self-made. A self-made man has seen hard-
ship and all that entails and then exorbitant wealth and what it can do for
him. He is therefore not too keen to part with his wealth. He wants to hoard
it. Mukesh Ambani's younger brother, Anil, has crashed from being a man
worth $40 billion to near bankruptcy, all because of business missteps.

Bill Gates and Warren Buffett have instituted a giving pledge, asking
the rich to donate at least half of their net income to philanthropy either
while living or when they pass away. As an aside, it surprises me that the
more Gates gives, the richer he becomes, but that's probably because Mi-
crosoft stock is doing so well. In 2011, Gates and Buffett traveled to India
to convince the country's superrich to give away their wealth. They did not
have much luck there. As of May 2019, the pledge has 204 signatories, but
looking down the list, I found only two from India, Azim Premji and Ki-
ran Mazumdar-Shaw. I ignored people of Indian origin, like Vinod Kho-
sla, who are based in the US and made their wealth there. A paltry two out
of 204 doesn't say much for Indian giving.

Perhaps the Tatas and the Birlas have for ages been doing their own
philanthropy, like building educational institutions and hospitals, and do
not feel the need for an alien hand like Bill Gates to guide them. And no
matter which way you spin it, Gates and Buffett get a lot of publicity out of
this initiative; it almost seems as if they are the ones doing all the giving,
which may not be to the liking of many rich people.

On March 28, Modi created the PM CARES Fund, which stands for
the Prime Minister's Citizen Assistance and Relief in Emergency Situa-
tions Fund. It's an ingenious description, but I don't like the angle of PM
CARES. It sounds too political to me. Modi asked everyone, big and
small, to help, with the minimum donation being fourteen cents. As of

May 15, over $400 million from this fund had been allocated for COVID relief.

This pandemic was supposed to see the dam burst for Indian giving. Bollywood megastar Akshay Kumar announced a donation of close to $14 million (in purchasing power parity terms) to the PM CARES fund.

Well, who am I to complain? Akshay is friends with the PM and put his millions into the fund. Azim Premji, who is incidentally a Muslim, and one of the two Indians on the Gates-Buffett pledge list, committed to donating over $500 million from his foundation. His company, Wipro, pledged to donate close to $70 million.

Hindu right-wing Muslim baiters leave people like Premji alone. They feel that he is a true patriot, as if it is up to them to decide who's a patriot and who's not. In the rarefied world of extreme wealth like Premji's, matters of religion lose importance. People like the Premjis can marry Hindus and no one will bat an eyelid in India. Such issues are meant only for the plebeians.

Ratan Tata, who heads the Tata Group, has pledged over $800 million. All of the figures here are in purchasing power parity terms. Mukesh Ambani has fished out about $275 million for the prime minister's relief fund. His company, Reliance, has also announced that it will set up a one-hundred-bed COVID-19 hospital in Mumbai. (When the virus arrived, India had 0.55 hospital beds per one thousand patients.)

Many other industrialists also have made substantial contributions. The first wave of COVID-19 has not hit India that hard in terms of an infection or fatality count. What it has done is displace hundreds of millions of migrant laborers who are going hungry. So, all the money that is making the PM's fund bulge is not going so much to tackling the disease as to feeding the poor and hungry. But starvation is an emergency, too, and many of those on the brink of starvation now are there because the lockdown left them stranded far from home and out of work.

But when the PM relaxes his lockdown, infections and deaths might spike. That's when India will need money for testing, tracing, and treatment, for more hospital beds and ventilators and personal protection equipment, such as masks and gowns. As social distancing recedes, the virus will expand its tentacles, and the expected second wave could be more furious than the first.

Pressure to ease his lockdown is on Modi as well. Even leaving the house for a walk has been banned. My friends in India tell me that they are going bonkers.

I have talked about Akshay, but no discussion of India will be complete without mentioning its other Bollywood superstar. Salman Khan, a Muslim, is arguably the biggest star in Bollywood. He was accused of driving drunk and crashing into a pavement dweller, killing him instantly. Khan fled the scene of the crime. As is usual in India, somebody else identified himself as the driver to the police. Usually, domestic help will pledge, having been promised enough compensation by their masters. The trial dragged on for years, and Khan, who, too, is close to Modi, was cleared of the hit-and-run case in 2015.

Salman Khan has many faults and has quite possibly done many crimes. But he has redeemed himself in the eyes of most of the public. Salman Khan has promised to feed twenty-five thousand film workers daily, but it is unclear for how long.

Shah Rukh Khan is another megastar, also a Muslim. He was unquestionably the number one star until Salman, arguably, displaced him from his perch. Shah Rukh announced that he will donate fifty thousand pieces of personal protection equipment. He said that he would feed fifty-five hundred families for a month in Mumbai. Shah Rukh will donate to the PM CARES relief fund, and he, along with his wife, will donate to the governor of the state of Maharashtra's relief fund.

Cricket is in India's blood. Sachin Tendulkar is India's biggest superstar. Tendulkar has decided to feed five thousand people for a month. He also donated about $300,000 for the fight against the epidemic. Other cricket stars followed suit.

The PM and the governors of various states better hoard their funds. One day or the other, calamitously or otherwise, the lockdown will end. Then the reverse migration of hundreds of millions of villagers to the cities will begin. There they will have to look for new accommodations, because their previous shanties would have been overtaken by local gang lords.

They will have to beg and plead with the rich and the middle classes for jobs that had either been done away with or furloughed without pay.

It's as if an entirely new economy will have to start up. India Inc. has thrived through crony capitalism and a captive domestic market. Exports of finished goods really have not been its forte. But the government will be almost bankrupt after this pandemic. It will not have large-scale contracts to dole out to its cronies. India's current GDP is about $3 trillion. Modi aspires to make it $5 trillion by 2024, which is when he is due to seek reelection.

Even before the pandemic, $5 trillion was proving a tall ask. Such a target amount would have required near double-digit growth in GDP. Modi was clocking only about half that. Now, $5 trillion seems like a pipe dream.

India Inc. and a lot of the rest of India's glitterati have emerged shining through this crisis. But what they have done is a drop in a country as vast as an ocean. At the best of times, they should have been following the Gates-Buffett 50 percent giving pledge. Now they will have to do much more. But giving fatigue is sure to set in. Until now, India has escaped the worst of the pandemic. But the pandemic promises to hover over the world like a black cloud for a year or two at least. India could yet met meet the fate of America and many countries of Europe. There's no letting one's guard down.

I would like to end on a positive note. Bill Gates has emerged as a philanthropist at large, a global savant. And the Gates Foundation in India is working with the government and its partners to eradicate the disease as well as reduce inequity. His commendations are treasured by kings and countries around the world. Here's what he just wrote Modi, praising his leadership in dealing with the coronavirus epidemic:

> "We commend your leadership and the proactive measures you and your government have taken to flatten the curve of the COVID-19 infection rate in India, such as adopting a national lockdown, expanding focused testing to identify hot spots for isolation, quarantining, and care, and significantly increasing health expenditures to strengthen the health system response and promote R&D and digital innovation.

"I'm glad your government is fully utilizing its exceptional digital capabilities in its COVID-19 response and has launched the Aarogya Setu digital app for coronavirus tracking, contact tracing, and to connect people to health services.

"Grateful to see that you're seeking to balance public health imperatives with the need to ensure adequate social protection for all Indians."

Pandit Jawaharlal Nehru was India's first prime minister. He was the foremost acolyte of Mahatma Gandhi. In a widely acclaimed speech delivered toward midnight of August 14, 1947 (India became independent on August 15, 1947), called "Tryst with Destiny," Nehru said this:

"The ambition of the greatest man of our generation has been to wipe every tear from every eye. That may be beyond us, but as long as there are tears and suffering, so long our work will not be over.

"Peace has been said to be indivisible; so is freedom, so is prosperity now, and so also is disaster in this one world that can no longer be split into isolated fragments.

"On this day our first thoughts go to the architect of this freedom, the father of our nation, who, embodying the old spirit of India, held aloft the torch of freedom and lighted up the darkness that surrounded us.

"We have often been unworthy followers of his and have strayed from his message, but not only we but succeeding generations will remember this message and bear the imprint in their hearts of this great son of India, magnificent in his faith and strength and courage and humility. We shall never allow that torch of freedom to be blown out, however high the wind or stormy the tempest."

Rather than a book with answers, this is a book that raises many questions. Has the lockdown helped India contain the virus? Will more people die of hunger than of the coronavirus in India? Will India forge an effective public health system? (At present, India spends only about 1.3 percent of its GDP on public health, among the lowest in the world.) Will the Indian economy rally and how? Perhaps the most baffling of all questions, is

India truly a positive outlier when it comes to the coronavirus? As oncologist Siddhartha Mukherjee has said, "To be totally frank, I don't know, and the world doesn't know the answer." He goes on to say that if we tested more, we would find the answer. It is time for the best Indian effort at jugaad. Finally, how will Modi fare?

For now, these are questions without answers. This is a work in progress. To be continued. As of Mother's Day 2020, there is a clear view of the Himalayas crowning the Delhi skyline—a view not seen in thirty years.

AFTERWORD

I am writing as of May 2020. The total number of reported infections in India is 106,886 and the number of deaths is 3,303. In deaths, this places India behind 15 countries including the US with 93,558 deaths, the UK with 35.341 deaths, China with 4,634 deaths, and Sweden with 3,743 deaths.

India is number seven in testing worldwide, with 2,512,388 tests. It lags behind the US which has conducted 12,647,099 tests and Russia which has conducted 7,500,000 tests. But on a tests-per-one-million-population basis, India has only 1,823 tests. The corresponding figure for the US is 38,234 and for Russia 51,395. The worldwide rank for India on a tests-per-one-million-population basis is 139. So, while India has fewer deaths than many other countries, testing is still a huge problem.

On April 13, 2020, the Supreme Court of India ordered that free tests for the coronavirus will be available only for the poorest, leaving the government to decide who else should get the benefit. The court had said the week before that free tests for COVID-19 should be available to all, but changed its decision after private laboratories expressed their inability to do so.

Private labs charge about Rs. 4,500 ($59) for the test. It's not cheap. The government of India issued an order on April 13 that it would reimburse private labs for testing the 500 million people covered by a flagship public health insurance scheme. The rest would have to pay.

As of May 2020, India is looking to double its coronavirus testing capacity to 100,000 per day, by increasing local production of test kits by the end of the month. The government recently announced it would no longer use Chinese-made kits, citing reliability problems.

"We will have indigenous production of good quality antibody kits, and also the RT-PCR kits for detection of the virus. I think all this is going to come in the next couple of weeks," stated Federal Health Minister Harsh Vardhan. Vardhan is set to take charge as chairman of the World Health Organization Executive Board on May 22. The main functions of the Executive Board are to give effect to the decisions and policies of the World Health Assembly, to advise it and to generally to facilitate its work.

Domestic production will also help to meet the target of conducting 100,000 tests a day by May 31, Vardhan said.

The RT-PCR, or reverse transcription polymerase chain reaction, a molecular probe that authorities call the "gold standard" test to detect the virus, is conducted by examining a sample from a nasal or throat swab. The results take up to eight hours to come back.

Prime Minister Modi has announced the fourth phase of his national lockdown. The lockdown was first imposed for twenty-one days starting March 25 and then extended on April 15 and later on May 4. Lockdown 3.0 ends on May 20. Modi's Lockdown 4.0 is set to begin on May 21, and last until May 31. There was some easing in Lockdown 3.0 with stand-alone shops lifting shutters and liquor shops opening up.

In Lockdown 4.0, Modi has given considerable flexibility to individual states for further relaxation. Inter-state movement of vehicles and buses has been allowed. Shops and markets can open with staggered timings. All shops will have to ensure six feet distance (2 *gaz ki doori*) among customers and cannot allow more than five people in at one time.

Now all we know for sure is what we don't know:

What happens to the virus as India reopens?
What happens to the Indian economy?
And what happens to Modi?

ACKNOWLEDGMENTS

Francis Leong, where would I be without you, my brother who means more than my blood brother to me? I want you to lead a long and healthy life so that we can grow old together.

Jaggi Kapur, keep playing golf and the other good stuff. You are ninety-three, and you are not leaving me until you hit a century.

I would like to express my gratitude to my superb editor, Meg Blackstone. My publisher, Arthur Klebanoff, is one of the most accomplished people that I have met. I am deep in debt to him and to his very fine team at RosettaBooks, which includes Brian Skulnik and Sara Brady, among many others.